D0871552

Sweet Surprise

A Scientific Approach

A Secret Weight Loss for Over 40

Hormone Balance

Stop Sugar and Refined Carb Cravings and Addiction

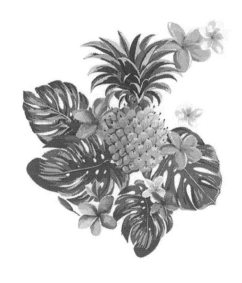

21 Days Sugar Detox to Boost Your Gut & Your Brain

by: Triya Redberg

© **Copyright Triya Redberg 2022 - All rights reserved.**

The content contained within this book may not be reproduced, duplicated, or transmitted without direct written permission from the author or the publisher.

Under no circumstances will any blame or legal responsibility be held against the publisher or author for any damages, reparation, or monetary loss because of the information contained within this book. Either directly or indirectly. You are responsible for your own choices, actions, and results.

ISBN: 979-8-9858689-0-6

Legal Notice:

This book is copyright protected. This book is only for personal use. You cannot amend, distribute, sell, use, quote, or paraphrase any part, or the content within this book, without the consent of the author or publisher.

Disclaimer Notice:

Please note the information contained within this document is for educational and entertainment purposes only. All effort has been executed to present accurate, up-to-date, and reliable, complete information. No warranties of any kind are declared or implied. Readers acknowledge that the author is not engaged in rendering legal, financial, medical, or professional advice. The content within this book has been derived from various sources. Please consult a licensed professional before attempting any techniques outlined in this book.

By reading this document, the reader agrees that under no circumstances is the author responsible for any losses, direct or indirect, which are incurred as a result of the use of the information contained within this document, including, but not limited to, — errors, omissions, or inaccuracies.

DEDICATION

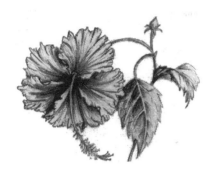

My dear father,

I wrote this book for you! You are in heaven now, and I want you to know that I'm so sorry that I spent little time listening and talking to you since I left home for school and work. It's too late to reclaim your life, but you motivate me every day to help so many lives.

I hear you, and I love you always!

Your little brown girl

TABLE OF CONTENTS

INTRODUCTION

ccording to the CDC, the number 1 leading cause of death in the USA is heart disease.[1] The World health organization (WHO) also has the same record. The number 1 leading cause of death globally is cardiovascular (heart disease and stroke).[2]

What are the risk factors of heart disease?

The answer is obesity, insulin resistance or diabetes, high cholesterol, and blood pressure.

Have you heard about metabolic syndrome?

A metabolic syndrome is a group of five conditions that can lead to heart disease, diabetes, stroke, and other health problems. Metabolic syndrome is diagnosed when someone has three or more risk factors:

1. High blood glucose (sugar)

2. Low levels of HDL ("good") cholesterol in the blood

3. High levels of triglycerides in the blood

4. Large waist circumference

5. High blood pressure

---

[1] Heart Disease | cdc.gov. (n.d.). CDC. https://www.cdc.gov/heartdisease/index.htm

[2] The top 10 causes of death. (2020, December 9). WHO | World Health Organization. https://www.who.int/news-room/fact-sheets/detail/the-top-10-causes-of-death

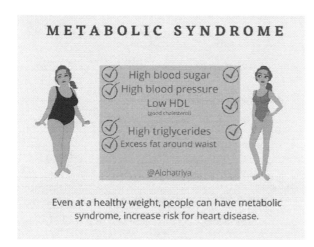

METABOLIC SYNDROME

High blood sugar
High blood pressure
Low HDL
(good cholesterol)
High triglycerides
Excess fat around waist

@Alchatriya

Even at a healthy weight, people can have metabolic syndrome, increase risk for heart disease.

Research in November 2021 showed up to 50% of the people who have died from COVID-19 had metabolic and vascular disorders.3

One-third of U.S. adults have metabolic syndrome, and it is increasing. Metabolic syndrome is linked to insulin resistance.4

Most people don't even know if they have insulin resistance, which happens worldwide because of our food every day.

The more technologies we have, the more problems arise. The food industry wants to increase the consumption of its products. But in the meantime, they want to lower the cost by using cheap and low-quality food even though it creates health issues. Sugar and refined

---

3 Steenblock, C., Schwarz, P., Ludwig, B., Linkermann, A., Zimmet, P., Kulebyakin, K., Tkachuk, V. A., Markov, A. G., Lehnert, H., de Angelis, M. H., Rietzsch, H., Rodionov, R. N., Khunti, K., Hopkins, D., Birkenfeld, A. L., Boehm, B., Holt, R., Skyler, J. S., DeVries, J. H., Renard, E., ... Bornstein, S. R. (2021). COVID-19 and metabolic disease: mechanisms and clinical management. The lancet. Diabetes & endocrinology, 9(11), 786–798. https://doi.org/10.1016/S2213-8587(21)00244-8

4 Saklayen M. G. (2018). The Global Epidemic of the Metabolic Syndrome. Current hypertension reports, 20(2), 12. https://doi.org/10.1007/s11906-018-0812-z

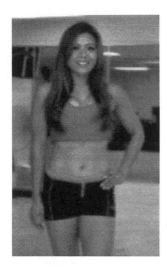

carbohydrates are one reason that leads to insulin resistance and metabolic syndrome.

I have been in the health and fitness industry as a personal trainer for over 15 years. I became a certified nutrition coach, specializing in blood sugar stabilization for more than ten years after my father passed away because of diabetes type 2 and heart disease.

I love my job, and it's a blessing. I help people change their path even before beginning the insulin resistance phase. Most people do not know if they have it, and some people come to me because they couldn't lose weight anymore, and some reason might relate to insulin resistance.

I focus on health & nutrition for people over-40s because I understand once you are over-40s, you might have some health complications, injuries, more stress, and hectic life with work and family. I'm also in my mid-40s, and I certainly understand people over-40s. Losing weight and keeping up with health is not easy for most. That's why you have me as your special someone who helps your life run smoother.

Detox for everyone is essential, especially if you have been in this body for a long time. Yes, 40 years is quite a long time. It is just like a car. If you have used the car for a long time, you need to change the oil and bring your vehicle to check up. Everyone has been exposed to chemicals that come with food, the environment, and everyday life products. So, it would help if you detox from time to time.

Another reason that most people can't lose weight is that their body is out of balance. Your body is intelligent but complicated. Once it's

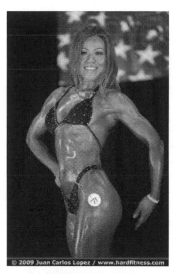

out of balance, it won't work. Your body might be out of balance because one or more of your body systems do not function as they should. You have 11 basic systems, and in this book, I emphasize the Endocrine System and hormones. Chapter 3 will show what hormones make you gain weight and what hormones help you lose weight.

© 2009 Juan Carlos Lopez / www.hardfitness.com

For those of you, pick up this book because you want to learn how to overcome sugar & refined carbohydrate cravings and addiction. You can discover this in chapter 4. It's not your fault that you have sugar & refined carbohydrates cravings or other addictions such as alcohol, drugs, and additional stimulation. You can blame your brain!

Even though I am a nutrition coach, a personal trainer, and a former bodybuilder who won NPC bodybuilding shows in Northern California. I fell for this trap too.

I went through my divorce in my late 30s until my early 40s. I gained a lot of weight because I didn't know the brain game and learned from any textbook before becoming a nutrition coach. I have learned about willpower, counting calories, and eating to control blood sugar and insulin to lose weight quickly during that time. It works for many of my clients and serves me until I have a significant shift in my life one day. I'm sure you have

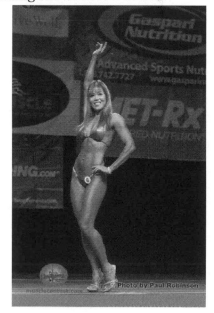

Photo by Paul Robinson

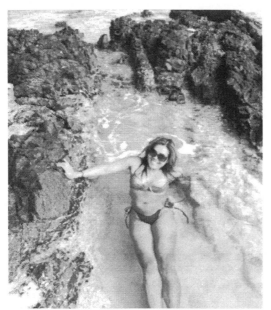

your own story too, and once that happens, you sink into the brain game that you don't know.

I also didn't recognize it because I was relying on calories in and calories out, exercising more and eating less, and willpower.

In 2017, I had an accident, slipped, and fell. I have had lower back and knee injuries, which have turned into chronic pain ever since. Even though I had knee surgery, my body wasn't the

same. I couldn't rely on exercise anymore because I couldn't even bend down to pick up my dog. Thank you, God, who showed me how to reclaim my health following the accident. I have always loved to read medical research related to nutrition and exercise. Fortunately, I found something that connected the dots of my addiction.

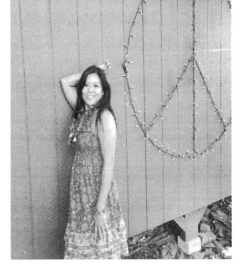

After divorce at the retreat center, Big Island, Hawaii

After my divorce, I had sugar, refined carbohydrate, and alcohol addiction. My fasting blood glucose and HbA1c were high. My cholesterol didn't look good at all. Yes, it was devastating because I am a nutrition coach, and where was my willpower? Today I also understood my father, who was slim, but why he had diabetes and heart disease. If you have sugar, refined carbohydrate, and alcohol addiction, you will have insulin resistance one day. Unless you stop it and it's not too late to take action today!

Two years after the accident, I have chronic pain and can't exercise like I used to, but I can get my healthy body back. My blood sugar and HbA1C are excellent. My HDL is outstanding (105), and my triglyceride is pretty low (45). I have learned and now better understand that the human body, mind, and spirit are connected as a masterpiece of creation.

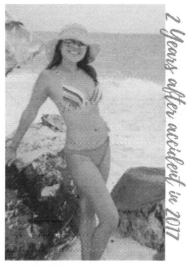

2 Years after accident in 2017

Chapter 1 to chapter 3 is basic information that I usually use to coach my clients—the simple details on food macronutrients, the differences of carbohydrates, losing weight by understanding our body systems, especially the endocrine system. When I do one-on-one coaching, I will look into the detail of each person because everyone is different and unique. But in chapters 1-3, it's only basic information.

Chapter 4 reveals how to overcome sugar and refined carb cravings and addiction with science-based strategies. I will show you step by step, and I'm sure it will help you.

Chapters 5,6 and 7. I spent a lot of time reading medical research, advancing nutrition science, and most nutrition publications as I do not believe in the media, internet, magazine, or even gurus that people follow, but in the end, they want to sell their supplements and products. It took time, but it's worth it. I will share the information with you in those chapters. Once you read it, you can forget about all the diets that confuse you.

Do you know about our brain chemistry? Serotonin is about 90% made in the gut, and over 50% of dopamine is made in the gut. In chapter 5, sugar detox with the gut microbiome principle will help you understand the link between the gut and the brain.

In chapter 6, I dive deep into this chapter with medical research. You will discover what causes gut dysbiosis and where we stand for 21 days sugar detox plan because what kills your gut microbiome will kill your brain, and, in the end, it will kill you.

Chapter 7 polyphenol-rich foods matter to your waistline and brain chemistry. You will explore polyphenol-rich foods that are not only grapes, berries, and wine but also other foods. The "sweet surprise" will help you open your eyes to the incredible information. You can use this information as a reference all year round. You won't see anyone put it all together as I do. Chapter 8 is the bonus for you.

Chapter 9 What is in and out in the 21 days sugar detox. It's a recap for you and especially those who didn't complete chapter 6 because it's too much information to digest in a short period, but you are excited to start the sugar detox ASAP.

I have a special gift for you at the end of the book. You can enter another book that I share with you, the meal plan and my secret for 21 days sugar detox. You may do only 7 days or 21 days detox, and it's up to you. You may not do the detox at all, but you use this book to guide your diet. No one can fool you for any diet from now on.

In the 7-day sugar detox, week 1, you will do liver, kidney, and gut detox at the same time. No counting calories, no confusion about glycemic index, glycemic load, and insulin index. I will show you the easy but accurate way. You may do it in week 2 and week 3 if you want more weight loss and have more benefits for your gut and your body systems.

Who should use the 21 days Sugar Detox?

- Everyone who wants to take your liver and kidney on vacation. Boost your gut microbiome, balance your hormones, and have better health. You are welcome to join the program if you are under the 40s too.

- If you want to drop 10 pounds in 2 weeks? If you are close to your standpoint, you will see a tiny waist and flat abdominal.

- Someone who wants to stop sugar & refined carbohydrate cravings and addiction.

- Everyone who prefers to improve their health wants to make sure you do not have insulin resistance, which causes metabolic syndrome.

- Someone wants to reverse diabetes type 2, lower blood glucose, lower HbA1C, lower triglyceride, lower blood pressure, increase HDL (good cholesterol) and enhance gut health.

- If you choose to harmonize your health and wellbeing,

- you seek vitality like 20 years old again.

- If you desire to look at least 10 years younger.

I make it simple, and it's easy to prepare even for men who don't know much about cooking.

The 21 days sugar detox plan has two levels:

Level 1 is for someone who has sugar & refined carbs cravings and food addiction. You regularly have soda, juice, sugar, refined carbohydrates, and sweets. Your everyday plate is not very healthy, but you want to make a change. You will start with week 2, follow week 3 and finish with week 1. You can repeat weeks 2 & 3 if you want to lose more weight or have better health and see improvement of your blood glucose, HbA1C or even reverse your type 2 diabetes and insulin resistance.

Level 2 is for someone who eats healthy over 80% of your daily consumption. You don't drink soda or have sugar, refined carbs, or any food addiction. You can start week 1, a level 2, right away. You can do the detox 2-3 times/year. (New year, spring and fall seasons), for week 2 & 3, you can use it as a part of your healthy eating year-round.

For the menu plan in week 1, only vegetarian, and in weeks 2 and 3, vegetarian and nonvegetarian.

My intention has been and continues to be to share the knowledge and practical approach to people on how to change the balance of food for better health, activities, and positive output to support people to be in balance and harmony, which can transform their life.

Aloha,

Triya

A Special Gift for You

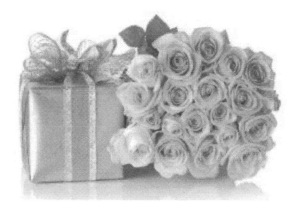

On the last page of the book

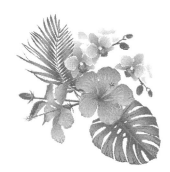

CHAPTER 1

WHAT IS SUGAR DETOX?

The first question that may cross your mind is,

DO I NEED A DETOX?

Let's see what detox is, according to the Merriam-webster dictionary.

The definition of "de": remove (a specified thing) from. [5]

The definition of "tox": poison[6]

We also can see "tox" is short of toxin, which means a poisonous substance that is a specific product of the metabolic activities of a living organism and is very unstable toxic when introduced into the tissues, and capable of inducing antibody formation.[7]

Definition of detox: detoxification from an intoxicating or addictive substance.

---

[5] DE Definition & Meaning. (n.d.). Merriam-Webster. Retrieved December 31, 2021, from https://www.merriam-webster.com/dictionary/DE

[6] Toxin Definition & Meaning. (n.d.). Merriam-Webster. Retrieved December 31, 2021, from https://www.merriam-webster.com/dictionary/toxin

[7] Toxin Definition & Meaning. (n.d.). Merriam-Webster. Retrieved December 31, 2021, from https://www.merriam-webster.com/dictionary/toxin

So now, let's review sugar.

IS SUGAR POISONOUS AND ADDICTIVE?

The answer is yes.

WHAT HAPPENS TO YOUR BODY WHEN YOU HAVE TOO MUCH SUGAR?

According to Robert Lustig, MD, a UCSF pediatric neuroendocrinologist. Said more Americans are overweight today than 30 years ago. Kids are still getting heavier compared with prior generations of kids. The problem is the increase in sugar consumption. Sugar drives fat storage and makes the brain think hungry, setting up a "vicious cycle."

It is fructose that is harmful, according to Lustig. Fructose is a part of the two most popular sugars. One is table sugar — sucrose. The other is high-fructose corn syrup. High-fructose corn syrup has become ubiquitous in soft drinks and many other processed foods. [1]

Since 1980, there has been growing concern about two new conditions linked to fructose consumption from added sugar and obesity and other unhealthy dietary additives, such as trans-fats:

First, Non-alcoholic fatty liver disease (NAFLD): excess fat build-up characterized this in the liver.

Second, Non-alcoholic steatohepatitis (NASH): fatty liver, a significant inflammation, and "steatosis," which is scarring as the liver tries to heal its injuries, characterizes this. That scarring cuts off vital blood flow to the liver. [2]

Sugar seems to have a significant impact on the body, directly and indirectly, leading to the development of metabolic syndrome.

So, what is metabolic syndrome? According to the World Health Organization, metabolic syndrome is a pathologic condition characterized by abdominal obesity, insulin resistance, high blood pressure, and a high concentration of lipids in the blood.

The most important thing to keep in mind is that metabolic syndrome, [3] sometimes referred to as syndrome X, is a group of metabolic abnormalities that occur in the same person. The conditions that most often arise are:

♦ Hyperglycemia: higher than average blood glucose or blood sugar levels, referred to as Hyperglycemia.

♦ Hypertension: When a person has hypertension, they have a condition where they have high blood pressure.

♦ Hyperlipidemia: a high-fat level in the blood and is often evidenced in high triglyceride levels and low in HDL (good cholesterol)

♦ Abdominal obesity: Excess fat around the abdomen or center of the body can leave a person in the abdominal obesity or overweight category. [4]

> **People with insulin resistance do not recognize if they have it. They usually have no symptoms at all. In most cases, insulin resistance isn't discovered until it gets serious with health issues.**

Now let's check your beauty and looks. You are in danger, too, if you have a sugar crush. Too much sugar affects not only your body organs but also your skin. Sugar intake affects your body by causing saggy skin, dark, patchy skin, wrinkled skin, rapid aging symptoms. The sugar we consume gets attached to the proteins in the bloodstream, and the phenomenon is called glycation. This process forms new molecular structures that damage skin elasticity, leading to skin aging.

Excess sugar consumption not only causes skin aging but also brain aging. Increased glucose and blood sugar levels deteriorate brain cells, negatively affecting memory power leading to cognitive impairment, which is also a dangerous way sugar affects your body.

Sugar can now lead to joint problems, too. According to science direct, Autoimmunity Reviews. High in refined carbohydrates and sugar and low in fiber and antioxidants might increase the risk of rheumatoid arthritis (RA) both directly through increasing inflammation and indirectly through increasing insulin resistance and obesity, with the latter being a known risk factor for RA. 5

How about your teeth? Sugar can ruin your teeth too. The American Journal of clinical nutrition showed that sugar destroys the healthy bacteria in your mouth, which can cause rotten teeth or bad oral health, causing plaque and cavities. 6

A HIGH-SUGAR DIET IMPACTS MENTAL HEALTH

Many studies have shown a sweet tooth's harmful effects on mood, learning, and quality of life. It may contribute to several mental health problems:

Addiction

Sugar and processed foods surge the brain with the feel-good chemical dopamine, which, over time, changes the function of the brain. In a study by researchers at Yale University, the simple vision of a milkshake activated the same reward centers of the brain as cocaine among people with addictive eating habits. A 2007 study showed that rats prefer sugar water to cocaine. Rats given fatty and sugary products showed classic symptoms of addiction, including tolerance and withdrawal symptoms when the products were taken away. 7

Depression

Sugar suppresses the activity of a hormone called BDNF that is low in individuals with depression and schizophrenia. Sugar is also at the root of chronic inflammation, which impacts the immune system, the brain, and other systems in the body; inflammation has also been implicated in depression. Interestingly, countries with high sugar intake also have a high rate of depression.

Anxiety

The high-sugar diet does not cause anxiety but worsens anxiety symptoms and impairs the body's ability to cope with stress. Individuals who suffer from panic attacks, for example, are hyper-alert to signs of impending danger. Sugar can cause blurry vision, difficulty thinking, and fatigue, all of which may be interpreted as signs of a panic attack, increasing worry and fear. A sugar high and later crash can cause shaking and tension, making anxiety worse.

Research has established a correlation between sugar intake and anxiety. In a 2008 study, rats that binged on sugar and then fasted displayed anxiety; in a 2009 study, rats fed sucrose compared to high-antioxidant honey were more likely to suffer anxiety. While dietary changes alone cannot cure anxiety, they can decrease symptoms, boost energy and improve the body's ability to cope with stress.

Learning and Memory

Sugar may also compromise cognitive abilities, such as learning and memory. In an animal study by researchers at the University of California, Los Angeles, six weeks of taking a fructose solution (like soda) caused the rats to forget their way out of a maze, since rats that ate a nutritious diet and those that consumed a high-fructose diet that also included omega-3 fatty acids found their way out faster. The high-sugar diet caused insulin resistance, damaging communications between brain cells that fuel learning and memory formation. [8]

The list of the harmful bittersweet goes on and on. You can also find more information from The University of California Television (UCTV) and check out "Sugar: The bitter truth" or "Learn the facts about sugar-how sugar impacts your health."

HOW MUCH IS TOO MUCH?

The American Heart Association (AHA) recommends only 6 teaspoons (25 grams) of added sugar per day for women and 9 teaspoons (38 grams) for men. The AHA limits for children vary depending on their age and caloric needs but range between 3-6 teaspoons (12 - 25 grams) per day.

That is in line with the World Health Organization (WHO) recommendation that only 10%–less–come from added sugar or natural sugars in honey, syrups, and fruit juice. For a 2,000-calorie diet, 5% would be 25 grams.

Sweet surprise

The average American consumes 17 teaspoons (71.14 grams) every day. That translates into about 57 pounds of added sugar consumed each year per person. [9]

Let's do the math!

Limit daily sugar to 6 tsp (25 g) for women, 9 tsp (38 g) for men.

1 teaspoon of sugar = 4.2 grams of sugar

1 can of Coca-Cola (12oz) = 39 grams of sugar = 9.2 teaspoons

1 Nutri-grain fruit and nut bar (100g) = 32.5 grams of sugar = 7.7 teaspoons

<u>*This is not a meal but a snack or a beverage between meals. Some people might drink more than a can of Coca-Cola per day.*</u>

Let's check out the typical American breakfast.

Cereal & milk and a cup of orange juice.

1 cup Kellogg's® Special K® Chocolate Delight Chocolate Cereal (Whole grain) = 13 grams of sugar

¾ cup skim milk = 22 grams of sugar

1 cup of orange juice = 20.83 grams of sugar Total sugar is 55.83 grams of sugar = 13.29 spoons of sugar

This is only breakfast. A cup of cereal isn't enough for some. We just pour it into a bowl because it's so convenient.

Everything is adding up from the salad dressing, ketchup, sauce, bread, frozen meal, low-fat yogurt, sports drink, granola, fruit juice, chocolate milk, iced tea, protein bar, vitamin water, pre-made soup, cereal bars, canned fruit, canned baked beans, pre-made smoothie, and the endless lists.

Let's take a tour with me. In the afternoon at Starbucks, I just want to grab a drink and a snack while meeting friends in town. I want only a tiny bit because I don't want to feel full before dinner. I order.

- *16 oz. Peppermint Mocha Frappuccino.*
- *A square of Dark Chocolate Fudge Brownie (54 g)*

Let's check the sugar content from nutrition facts.

16 oz. Peppermint Mocha Frappuccino = sugars 64 g.

A square of Dark Chocolate Fudge Brownie = sugars 19 g

Oh! My god. It's 83 grams of sugar, equal to 19.7 spoons of sugar. I just wanted a quick bite, but it turned out to be a complete disaster.

Consuming too much-added sugar over long periods also can affect the natural balance of hormones that drive critical functions in the body. Eating sugar increases glucose levels in the bloodstream, which leads the pancreas to release insulin. Higher insulin levels cause the body to store more food calories as fat.

Insulin also affects a hormone called leptin, our natural appetite suppressant that tells our brains we are full and can't stop eating. Imbalanced insulin levels and high consumption of certain sugars, such as fructose, have been linked to a condition called leptin resistance, in which the brain no longer hears the message to stop eating, thus promoting weight gain and obesity.

Leptin resistance enabled our ancestors to survive prolonged periods of the limited food supply by encouraging them to overeat during times of plenty and allowing them to conserve more calories as fat. It isn't a benefit in the modern world. To make matters worse, people with leptin resistance also felt sluggish, making it challenge to be active and contributing to further weight gain.

You can also view "The Truth About Sugar - New Documentary 2015" made by Science Fiction Documentary from a YouTube video.

QUIZ: DO YOU NEED A SUGAR DETOX?

Checklist

1. Do you have mood swings?

2. Are you craving sweets or refined carbohydrates?

3. Do you feel sluggish?

4. Do you have anxiety?

5. Do you have a poor memory?

6. Do you have insomnia?

7. Do you have a hormone imbalance?

8. Do you feel irritable?

9. Do you have food allergies?

10. Do you have a Foggy brain?

11. Do you feel fatigued?

12. Do you have depression?

13. Do you have infertility or decreased sex drive?

14. Do you have skin breakouts?

15. Do you have skin and nail infections?

16. Do you have digestive tract issues? Diarrhea, constipation, or bloating?

17. Are you overweight (Body mass index or BMI over 25)? Go to https://www.nhlbi.nih.gov/health/educational/lose_wt/BMI/bmicalc.htm

18. Do you have extra belly fat? Your waist circumference is greater than 35 inches for women or greater than 40 inches for men.

19. Do you have trouble losing weight?

20. Do you have high blood pressure?

21. Do you have high levels of triglycerides (over 100 mg/dl) or low HDL cholesterol (under 50 mg/dl)?

22. Do you have heart disease?

23. Is your fasting blood sugar greater than 100 mg/dl?

24. Have you been diagnosed with insulin resistance, pre-diabetes, or diabetes?

25. Is your hemoglobin A1c level greater than 5.7%?

26. Do you think about dessert or sweets even if you are not hungry?

27. Do you crash in the afternoon every day and look for something sweet to drink or eat to help?

28. You can't get through the day without sugar in your soft drink, coffee/tea, or some energy drink?

29. Are you unable to celebrate a birthday or other event without dessert or something sweet?

Suppose you answer yes to over 5 of the above questions. You should know that those are sugar overload symptoms. You should start the sugar detox program as soon as you can.

"If you don't sacrifice for what you want,

what you want becomes the sacrifice."

— *Anonymous*

HOW CAN THE SUGAR DETOX HELP YOU?

Suppose you have sugar overload symptoms or chronic health issues such as obesity, cardiovascular disease, hypertension, diabetes, or insulin resistance. The sugar detox can help you. Most people with diabetes don't know they have it until a symptom appears. Don't let it get that far. Start eating the right way now.

Following the sugar detox plan will help you reverse your chronic health problems, such as diabetes, insulin resistance, cardiovascular disease, and obesity. You will feel better after having your meals. Your problem with fatigue, mood swings, anxiety, depression, weight gain, and other sugar overload symptoms would be solved. You will have more energy during the day, and you will look younger at the bonus point.

The sugar detox plan is a whole foods regimen that is the best for improving health and preventing disease. Whole foods—like vegetables, fruits, whole grains, nuts, and legumes -keep their fiber and the entire portfolio of beneficial phytochemicals and micronutrients often removed in processed foods. You will have more energy and lose body fat, which will cause overall weight loss and better health. The sugar detox plan also stabilized your blood sugar with meals that combined the right amount of carbohydrate, protein, and fat, resulting in higher satiety and reduced cravings for sugar and carbohydrate.

TO-DO-LIST

1. Get a blood test

    Recommendation.

- A complete blood count (CBC)

- Hemoglobin A1C

- Comprehensive metabolic profile (blood glucose, calcium, and electrolyte tests, as well as blood tests that measure kidney function and liver function)

- Lipoprotein panel (check levels of LDL and HDL cholesterol and triglycerides in your blood)

2. Check your Body Mass Index (BMI)

3. Start cutting out soda (if you drink) and anything with "high fructose corn syrup" (HFCS).

"Your body can stand almost anything.

It's your mind that you have to convince."

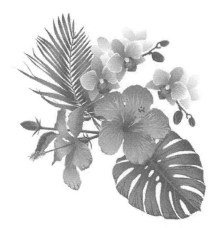

CHAPTER 2

THE TRUTH ABOUT

CARBOHYDRATES

WHAT IS A CARBOHYDRATE?

My clients always ask me about carbohydrates, short for "carbs." Can I eat carbs if I want to drop weight? Do carbs make me fat? Can I eat fruit? What carbs can I have? And what diet is best? Low carbs such as Paleo, Atkins, or even Keto diet. The fact is diet won't last for long, but it might help you for rapid weight loss, and they are not healthy in the long run.

Carbs are not bad because your body needs carbs for energy, and don't forget that your brain also needs carbs. But consuming too many carbs or the wrong types of carbs is the problem. Your blood sugar swings like a roller coaster because of insulin release once you eat the wrong kind of carbs or a big load of carbs. Therefore, learning about what is suitable for you will be beneficial for you to monitor your blood sugar, resulting in weight loss and solving chronic health problems.

A carbohydrate is one of three types of food that gives your body energy. The other two are proteins and fats. Together, they provide the fuel your body uses to build and repair itself. Carbs break down into glucose (sugar) that you can use right away. Carbs are found in vegetables, fruits, dairy, and grains - foods comprise starches, sugar, and fiber. Your body runs on glucose. Your brain needs it to work the way it should. Carbohydrates are an almost instant source of it. Your body can use fat for specific needs, but not all of them. Plus, fat used for fuel makes compounds called ketones that can raise the acid level in your blood, which can be unhealthy over the long term. 10

Carbs have the most significant impact on your blood sugar and insulin. If you want to know how many carbohydrates you need daily, think how much you need to use daily for physical activities and exercise. I want you to think about your car; how much gas you need when you drive from San Francisco to Berkeley (13.6 miles) vs. from San Francisco to Los Angeles (381.6 miles). You require more gas when you go a long distance, and it's a similar scenario with your body. Your body needs more energy when you have more physical activities. Consuming more carbs than your body needs daily leads you to gain weight, release insulin hormones, and store fat.

HOW ARE CARBOHYDRATES METABOLIZED IN THE BODY?

During digestion, carbohydrates are broken down into simple, soluble sugars that can be shipped across the intestinal wall into the circulatory system to be transported throughout the body. Carbohydrate digestion begins in the mouth with the action of salivary amylase on starches. It ends with monosaccharides being absorbed across the epithelium of the small intestine once the absorbed monosaccharides are sent to the tissues. (Monosaccharides are the simplest types of sugar. They build disaccharides and polysaccharides. Glucose, fructose, and galactose are examples of monosaccharides). Glucose or blood sugar is stored as glycogen in your muscles and liver, and your body draws on this for short-term energy. Eighty percent of the remaining glucose goes into the bloodstream for use by the cell in your body. If the leftover glucose is more than what the liver can hold, it can turn into fat storage for use later. Fructose, a sugar found in fruits and sugar added as high fructose corn syrup, such as processed food or soda, is metabolized through your liver, converted to fat, and stored for later use.

For this reason, please pay close attention to high fructose corn syrup and many processed foods that contain fructose because it's easy to convert to fat and leads to non-alcoholic fatty liver disease (NAFLD) and non-alcoholic steatohepatitis (NASH).

It would be best to have glucose to power cells throughout your systems. Since glucose from carbohydrates is the primary energy source throughout your body. Your systems need them at regular intervals to use for fuel. [11]

WHAT IS THE DIFFERENCE BETWEEN CARBOHYDRATES AND SUGAR?

First, I would like to introduce you to carbohydrates. Did you know there are three main types of carbohydrates in food?

First, starches. Second, sugars and third fibers.

You may have heard about "added sugar," "complex carbohydrate," "refined grains," and "whole grains," "sugar alcohol," "low-calorie sweeteners," "enriched grains," and the lists go on and on.

We live in a society that makes us confused since we have high technologies, and more food consumption options. If we wish to have a positive aspect of life, we should simplify it. I want to present you with a simple method of success.

Starches

Have you ever noticed someone with so much energy you wish you could bottle it for yourself? Plants have their way of 'bottling' energy. They do this by storing energy as starch. But what is starch? Starch is long chains of sugar molecules linked like a chain. A single sugar molecule is a monosaccharide.

Many sugar molecules linked are polysaccharides. Starch, therefore, is a polysaccharide or larger carbohydrate. (Main 5 types of polysaccharides are starch, dextrin, cellulose, pectin, and glycogen) [12]

Remember "Poly" ---> Many

Food High in starch include

1. Starchy vegetables, such as beans (kidney, navy, pinto, black-eyed peas, split peas, cannellini), butternut squash, chickpeas, corn, lentils, parsnips, peas, potatoes, sweet potatoes, taro, and yams.

2. Whole grains, such as barley, oats, rice, rye, spelt, teff, triticale, wheat, wild rice, millet, quinoa, amaranth, buckwheat, chia, and sorghum.

3. Processed grains, such as bread, pasta, noodle, crackers, cereals, and pastries.

Sugar

Sugar is another type of carbohydrate. There are two main types of sugar. The first is sugar, such as the lactose in milk or fructose in fruit. The second one is adding sugar, which is added during processing—for example, high-fructose corn syrup or brown rice syrup.

SUGARS, BROKEN DOWN

MONOSACCHARIDES (one-molecule sugar)

Remember "Mono" ---> One (1)

1. Glucose (All other carbohydrates and all other sugars are converted to glucose within the digestive system)

2. Fructose (levulose or fruit sugar and honey)

3. Galactose (occurs in milk)

DISACCHARIDES (two monosaccharides joined)

Remember "Di" ---> two (2)

1. Sucrose (table sugar) = glucose + fructose,

   For example, sugar cane and sugar beet

2. Lactose (milk sugar) = glucose + galactose

3. Maltose (malt sugar) = glucose + glucose.

You can recognize other sugars on labels because their chemical names also end in "-ose."

You can find sugar in different forms and nicknames. According to Dr. Lustig's sugar has 56 other names. [13]

FIFTY-SIX NAMES FOR SUGAR:

1. Agave nectar*

2. Barbados sugar*

3. Barley malt

4. Beet sugar*

5. Blackstrap molasses*

6. Brown rice syrup*

7. Brown sugar*

8. Buttered syrup*

9. Cane juice crystals*

10. Cane sugar*

11. Caramel*

12. Carob syrup*

13. Castor sugar*

14. Confectioner's sugar*

15. Corn syrup

16. Corn syrup solids

17. Crystalline fructose

18. Date sugar*

19. Demerara sugar*

20. Dextran

21. Dextrose

22. Diastatic malt

23. Diastase

24. Ethyl maltol

25. Evaporated cane juice*

26. Florida crystals*

27. Fructose*

28. Fruit juice*

29. Fruit juice concentrate*

30. Galactose

31. Glucose

32. Glucose solids

33. Golden sugar*

34. Golden syrup*

35. Grape sugar*

36. High-fructose corn syrup*

37. Honey*

38. Icing sugar*

39. Invert sugar*

40. Lactose

41. Malt syrup

42. Maltose

43. Maple syrup*

44. Molasses*

45. Muscovado sugar*

46. Organic raw sugar*

47. Panocha*

48. Raw sugar*

49. Refiner's syrup*

50. Rice syrup

51. Sorghum syrup*

52. Sucrose*

53. Sugar*

54. Treacle*

55. Turbinado sugar*

56. Yellow sugar*

* Contains fructose

Fiber

Fiber is the general name for specific carbohydrates — parts of vegetables, plants, and grains — that the body can't digest. While fiber isn't broken down and absorbed like nutrients, it still plays a crucial role in good health. Fiber contributes to digestive health, helps to keep your bowel movement regular, and makes you satisfied and feel full with your meals.

There are two main types of fiber. They are soluble fiber (which dissolves in water) and insoluble fiber (which does not dissolve in water). Combined, they're called total fiber.

Insoluble fiber adds bulk to stools. It helps treat constipation and diverticular disease and may benefit people with some types of IBS (irritable bowel syndrome). Recent research has shown that increased fiber is also linked to improved survival in people with colon cancer.

Soluble fiber is found in lentils, beans, peas, oatmeal, oat bran, nuts, seeds, psyllium, blueberries, pears, strawberries, and apples. Soluble fiber seems to lower cholesterol levels. It binds with cholesterol in the intestines and prevents it from being absorbed. It can slow the absorption of carbohydrates, helping to improve blood sugar levels. Soluble fiber may also be useful in treating diabetes and insulin resistance (prediabetes).

Insoluble fiber is found in brown rice, whole grains, barley, whole-grain couscous, bulgur, wheat bran, nuts, seeds, carrots, cucumbers, zucchini, celery, green beans, dark leafy vegetables, raisins, nuts, grapes, and tomatoes. 14

What are Daily fiber recommendations?

According to the Institute of Medicine, women need 25 grams of fiber per day, and men need 38 grams per day. Most Americans do not consume enough fiber in their diet. It's a brilliant idea to aim for this goal. Any increase in fiber in your diet can be beneficial. Eating more plant foods, vegetables, fruit, beans, whole grains, and nuts is the best way to increase your fiber intake.

GOOD CARBS VS. BAD CARBS

Not all carbs are created equal. The way carbs are broken down in our body makes carbs more or less preferred. Some carbs break down quickly, and it raises your blood sugar rapidly, and you want to avoid this type of carbs. Some carbs take longer to break down, and some don't digest like fibers. Do you wonder why?

You can find carbohydrates in almost every food in your diet. They include rice, pasta, noodle, bread, fruit, vegetables, and dairy products. They also have processed foods, such as frozen, packaged foods, snacks, beverage drinks, and fast food, filled with sugar, fat, and preservatives.

Whole foods represent foods that keep their natural composition and contain no artificial additives or preservatives. Whole foods contain vitamins, minerals, water, fiber, fatty acids, amino acids, carbohydrates, and much more. This is a more desirable carbohydrate to consume because it takes longer to digest. These include the starches found in whole-grain foods, vegetables, and beans. Since starches take longer to metabolize than sugar, they have a time-release energy effect. They will raise your blood sugar slowly and offer more sustained energy levels.

Processed foods are defined as foods that have been removed from their natural state because of chemical, biological, and mechanical manipulation. If food has been highly processed-meaning many of its nutrients have been stripped- it will quickly turn into sugar in the body. When it happens, the glucose will enter your bloodstream rapidly, causing a spike in blood sugar, which leads to a subsequent crash that can trigger hunger and lead to food cravings. If you consume a large number of carbs, it will lead to a significant rise in blood sugar, which will then cause your body to produce insulin. Suppose you repeat this cycle over and over again. In that case, you will end up with insulin resistance, which is a precursor to diabetes.

Bad Carbs - Ultra-processed carbs

(Say NO To these)

Processed food has a poor reputation as a diet saboteur. It's blamed for obesity rates, high blood pressure, and the rise of Type 2 diabetes.

Not all processed foods are created equal. Not all processed food is unhealthy. When we dive into the nitty-gritty of it, there are plenty of processed foods that can be a very healthy addition to your diet.

THE TRICK IS KNOWING WHICH FOODS TO AVOID.

According to the World, Public Health Nutrition Association helps define these different food processing levels. 15 They are defined into these four groups:

1. Minimally processed foods.

Think whole foods like fruits, veggies, meat, and nuts. Freezing, vacuum-sealing, and similar methods to preserve shelf life are acceptable here.

2. Processed Ingredients

The next level of processing is obtained or extracted from the whole foods in group one. Think: sugar and molasses got from cane or beets, honey extracted from the honeycomb, canned coconut milk, and oils made from nuts or fruits, like olive oil. These items may contain additives to preserve freshness.

3.   Processed Foods

These processed foods contain just two or three ingredients. Think: tuna jarred in olive oil, canned veggies, salted and packed nuts, boxed almond milk, and cured or smoked meats. Beer, wine, and ciders also fall here because they contain over one ingredient and are processed from whole foods like grapes or barley.

4.   Ultra-Processed

This is the mega-processed group of foods. They often include artificial colors, dyes and additives, non-sugar sweeteners, and processing aids such as caking and glazing agents, emulsifiers, and humectants. Examples of typical ultra-processed products are carbonated drinks; sweet or savory packaged snacks; ice-cream, chocolate, candies (confectionery); mass-produced packaged; bread and buns; margarine and spreads; cookies (biscuits), pastries, cakes, and cake mixes; breakfast 'cereals,' 'cereal' and 'energy' bars; 'energy' drinks; milk drinks, 'fruit' yogurts and 'fruit' drinks; cocoa drinks; meat and chicken extracts and 'instant' sauces; infant formulas, follow-on milk, other baby products; 'health' and 'slimming' products such as powdered or 'fortified' meal and dish substitutes; and many ready to heat products including pre-prepared pies and pasta and pizza dishes; poultry and fish 'nuggets' and 'sticks,' sausages, burgers, hot dogs, and other reconstituted meat products, and powdered and packaged 'instant' soups, noodles, and desserts.

The ideal diet avoids Group 4 entirely. The more processing that occurs, the less healthy the food becomes. Consuming too many calories from these foods results in obesity, blood sugar issues, and other metabolic diseases.

However, groups one to three are more of a gray area.

HERE ARE A FEW OTHER TIPS FOR CHOOSING PROCESSED FOOD

1. Whole foods or extracts from whole foods (like olive oil, coconut oil) should make up most of the ingredient list.

2. Preservatives should be natural. Look for vitamin E instead of chemical compounds like polysorbate 80 and sodium nitrate.

3. Choose glass-packaged foods over canned or plastic-wrapped foods since these can leach toxins into the food.

4. If you see "refined" in the ingredients, do not buy it.

5. Like fresh foods, choose wild-caught, grass-fed, and organic.

6. Choose preservatives in water or olive oil instead of vegetable oil.

7. Choose low sodium—for example, canned tomato products or nut products.

Good Carbs - The more nutritious carbohydrates (Choose these)

The best carbohydrate choice is "Whole Foods." The food comes from mother earth. Whole foods are as nature-made them are, without added fat, sugar, or sodium. They are rich in fiber and high in micronutrients, including vitamins and minerals and chemicals found in plants called phytonutrients. Everyone needs to consume micronutrients because they have many essential roles in the functioning of the body and brain.

Here are the best choices of carbohydrate foods:

1. Non-Starchy vegetables

First, leafy greens like spinach, kale, Swiss chard, and lettuce

Second, cruciferous vegetables like cauliflower, broccoli, Brussels sprouts, and cabbage

2. Starchy vegetable

First, summer squash like zucchini, Calabacitas (Mexican gray), and yellow squash.

Second, winter squash like pumpkin, butternut squash, and spaghetti squash

Third, root vegetables like sweet potatoes, burdock, beets, and parsnips

3. Fruits

First, berries like blueberries, raspberries, strawberries, acai, and goji berries.

Second, citrus fruits like oranges, grapefruit, lemons, and limes.

Third, others such as apples, avocados, tomatoes.

4. Nuts & Seeds

Nuts like walnuts, Brazil nuts, pecans, and cashews

Seeds like pepitas, flax seeds, hemp seeds, chia seeds, and sunflower seeds.

5. Legumes

- Beans like chickpeas, black beans, lima beans, and white beans

- Lentils (including green, red, yellow, and black)

- Peas (including snap, green, split, and snow)

6. Whole Grains

Whole grains are those that haven't been stripped, separated, or otherwise processed. Whole grains are a much more nutritious choice than refined grains. Do you wonder what the difference is?

All grains contain three parts:

First, bran is the hard outer shell of the grains. It is the part of the grain that provides the most fiber and most of the B vitamins and minerals.

Second, the Endosperm is the soft part of the center of the grain. It contains starch.

Third, the germ is the seed for a new plant within the grain and is packed with nutrients, including healthy fat and vitamin E.

"Whole grain" means that all three parts of the grain kernel are in the food, so you get all the nutrients that the grain offers. Most refined grains, such as white bread and white rice, have had the most nutritious part of the kernel (the bran and germ) removed during the processing. So, you only get the Endosperm of the starchy part of the grains, causing you to miss out on a lot of vitamins, minerals, and fiber.

Avoid any grains with gluten, like wheat, because they cause issues for many people.

Gluten-Free Whole grains are brown, black, and wild rice, oats*, buckwheat, millet, quinoa, teff, sorghum, corn, amaranth, and montina (Indian rice grass)

*Note oats:

Oats are gluten-free but are frequently contaminated with wheat during growing or processing. Several companies such as Bob's Red Mill, Cream Hill Estates, GF Harvest (formerly Gluten-Free Oats), Montana Gluten-Free, and Avena Foods are among those that are over pure, uncontaminated oats. 16

Whole foods offer many health benefits, such as enhancing overall nutrition, promoting gut health, supporting the immune system, protecting your heart, keeping blood sugar stabilized, and helping you to look younger. Nothing will go wrong once you eat the food from the sources. Eat live food, and you will be alive.

TO-DO-LIST

1. Gradually increase the fiber in your diet until you reach 25-35 grams per day by eating more vegetables and fruits.

2. Cut out all refined products and all ultra-processed food.

3. Start getting rid of foods with over 10 grams of sugar per serving.

4. Adding outdoor activities such as walking, hiking, walking dogs, or walking with friends and family.

5. Smile more often.

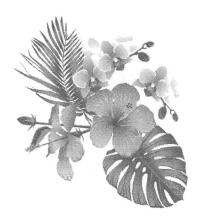

CHAPTER 3

WHAT MAKES YOU STORE FAT?

If you wish to have something work better for you, you need to understand how to run it properly. For example, you just bought a brand-new iPhone. So, you need to understand each feature, button, set up, how to operate it, how to make it work better, and troubleshoot once it breaks. Everything in the universe is just like the iPhone. We need to learn what it is and understand how to keep it in the best working condition. It's like a human body. If you want it to work better. You need to understand its function and learn how to have it work. Run better and wiser by understanding it. You can turn into an expert whenever you can't troubleshoot the problem by yourself, or you want to save your time and energy. When I can't fix my phone issue, I will call Apple customer support to help.

THREE IMPORTANT HORMONES THAT MAKE YOU STORE FAT

1. Insulin

2. Cortisol

3. Female hormones (estrogen and progesterone)

In this book, we will talk about insulin and cortisol only. Estrogen and progesterone will be in another book because this is a long topic for explaining and solving a problem for women over 40. You might control your body weight by knowing the secret of hormones insulin and cortisol, and by then, the estrogen hormone won't bother you when you have menopause.

EIGHT HORMONES HELP YOU MELT FAT

1. Growth hormones (GH)

2. Glucagon

3. Testosterone

4. Thyroid hormones (T3 and T4)

5. Insulin-like growth factor (IGF)

6. Adrenal

7. Melatonin

8. Leptin & Ghrelin [17]

WHAT IS INSULIN?

Insulin is released from the beta cells in your pancreas in response to rising glucose in your bloodstream. Insulin lowers blood sugar levels and stimulates glucose, protein, and fat metabolism. Insulin stores nutrients right after the meal. It stimulates the liver and muscle cells to store glucose as glycogen. It stimulates fat cells to make fats from fatty acids and glycerol. Insulin works with insulin-like growth factor (IGF) and glucagon to keep fuel constant in the blood, so when IGF and glucagon go down, insulin must go up. In the presence of insulin, you cannot burn fat. Sugar and refined carbohydrates trigger insulin. Large amounts of protein can produce insulin as well. 50–60% of protein becomes glucose. [18]

THE FIRST KEY; STOP STORING FAT

So, if you don't want to store fat, the best way to do so is trying not to trigger insulin by eating the right combination of the food each meal, which I'm going to guide you on this plan. Also, take a note that eating triggers insulin. That's why eating less often, or intermittent fasting is the best way not to store fat. I have a significant result with intermittent fasting, and I can share it with you in the future. In this book, you will focus on 21 days of sugar detox to help you lose weight, regain your health, stop sugar and refined carb cravings, and overcome sugar addiction. However, combining with intermittent fasting would benefit you because fasting leads to a significant increase in Human Growth Hormones (HGH) levels. Suppose you want to do intermittent fasting with 21 days of sugar detox. In that case, I recommend the 16/8 intermittent fasting for a good start. If you are not familiar with fasting, you simply do 12/12. You have your dinner at 7 pm. And go to sleep once you wake up, then have your breakfast at 7 am. It's simple. After that, you can extend the time to be 14 hrs. And the next 16 hrs. And now you got it—16/8 intermittent fasting.

WHAT IS INSULIN RESISTANCE?

Insulin resistance is when your muscles, fat, and liver don't respond well to insulin and can't take glucose from your blood. As a result, your pancreas makes more insulin to help glucose enter your cells. It's just like when you try to talk to a deaf person. Raise your voice so the deaf can hear you. Once this happens over time, your blood sugar levels go up more and more every day until it won't respond anymore, and you store more fat when it happens. [19]

Both insulin resistance and metabolic syndrome are powerful risk factors for developing cardiovascular disease and type 2 diabetes (T2D)[20]

WHAT IS PRE-DIABETES?

Pre-diabetes means your blood sugar levels are higher than usual but not high enough to be diagnosed with diabetes. Pre-diabetes occurs in people who already have some insulin resistance or whose beta cells in the pancreas aren't making enough insulin to keep blood glucose in the normal range. Extra glucose stays in your bloodstream rather than entering your cells without enough insulin. Over time, you could develop type 2 diabetes. [21]

Sweet surprise

The record in 2020.

❖ *Over 88 million people aged 18 and older have pre-diabetes (34.5% of the adult US population)*

❖ *Total: 34.2 million people have diabetes. (10.5% of the US population)* [22]

❖ *More than 4.9 million people in the UK have diabetes.*

❖ *13.6 million people are now at increased risk of type 2 diabetes in the UK.*

❖ *850,000 people in the UK live with type 2 diabetes but are yet to be diagnosed.* [23]

Insulin resistance and pre-diabetes usually have no symptoms. If you're older than 45, you should take a test. Doctors use blood tests to determine if someone has pre-diabetes, but they don't test for insulin resistance. Doctors often use the fasting plasma glucose (FPG) test or the A1C test to diagnose pre-diabetes. Some doctors also use the Oral Glucose Tolerance Test (OGTT), a two-hour test that checks your blood sugar levels before and two hours after you drink a special sweet drink. It tells the doctor how your body processes sugar.

HOW DO YOU KNOW IF YOU HAVE PRE-DIABETES?

Results showing pre-diabetes are:

An A1C of 5.7%–6.4%

Fasting blood sugar of 100–125 mg/dl

An OGTT 2-hour blood sugar of 140 mg/dl–199 mg/dl [24]

WHAT SPIKES INSULIN?

1. High fructose corn syrup, sugar, hidden sugars.

2. Refined carbohydrates.

3. MSG and hidden MSG (modified food starch)

4. Frequency meals (snack)

5. Stress (cortisol)

6. Large amounts of protein are eaten in a meal.

7. Alcohol

WHAT CAUSES INSULIN RESISTANCE?

Most people's answer is sugar and carbohydrates. The answer will shock you because fat causes insulin resistance; however, sugar makes you store more fat. Even though fat doesn't spike blood sugar, fat is a root cause of insulin resistance. You might not believe it because everyone knows that sugar and carbohydrates spike blood sugar, but that isn't all true. It won't spike your blood sugar if you have good carbs, as you read in chapter 2, and carbs with fiber. You can see the vegetarians who consume whole food plant-based diet have a lean and healthy body even though they consume a lot of carbohydrates. However, not all vegetarians have a slim and healthy body. If you consume vegetarian food, but it's not a whole food plant-based diet, you can gain more weight and have some health problems. 25

> *Sweet surprise*
>
> *Carbs don't cause type 2 diabetes or insulin resistance. The root cause of type 2 diabetes is insulin receptors that don't work correctly. Therefore, sugar and the blood couldn't get into the cell and accumulate and cause damage to the organs.*

Simply avoiding carbohydrates and taking medications are great ways to manage your diabetes. Still, it doesn't get to the root cause of type 2 diabetes. To get to the root cause of type 2 diabetes, we have to make the insulin receptor work again. Once the insulin receptor works again, you can eat carbohydrates without worrying that blood sugar is going high. That is a major goal to treat type 2 diabetes. Many kinds of research have shown the related "Intramyocellular Lipid, "insulin resistance, and type 2 diabetes. 26

Let's look at what happens after we eat. Our digestive tract breaks down into glucose, amino acids, and fatty acids when we eat food. The simple sugars are absorbed into our bloodstream and go to the cell, where they are taken up with the help of insulin and insulin receptors to the cells. Inside the cell, the sugar turns into ATP, which is energy. With type 2 diabetes, there is plenty of insulin around, but the insulin doesn't work because a lock is gummed up, so sugar can't get inside the cell. What causes the key to gum up? It's fat, also known as intramyocellular lipid in our muscle or intrahepatic cellular in our liver cells. The fat build-up in these cells means it gummed the insulin receptor up and that the channel which allows sugar to get in simply does not open. Therefore, it doesn't matter how much insulin is in our blood; the sugar can't get it. Your body responds by producing more insulin, and that may function temporarily. Still, the pancreas can become tired of making so much insulin over time. The insulin receptors get more and more jammed. Sugar builds up outside the cell, and you may be diagnosed with diabetes. 27

> ### Sweet surprise
>
> The key to treating type 2 diabetes is not to cut the amount of sugar in your bloodstream; the key is to make those insulin receptors work again by getting rid of the fat inside the cells.

From study has shown to improve insulin sensitivity and linked to metabolic abnormalities by reducing dietary saturated fat, replaced by monounsaturated and polyunsaturated fats. Therefore, the low carb and high fat, i.e., keto diet, just blind the problem. Still, it doesn't help the root cause, especially with saturated fat from animals.

In this sugar detox program, you will have a whole food plant-based diet with a good amount of fat from plant-based and omega-3.

NEXT HORMONE THAT MAKES YOU STORE FAT?

The answer is cortisol.

What is cortisol?

Cortisol is often called the "stress hormone" because of its relation to the stress response. However, cortisol is much more than just a hormone released during stress.

Cortisol is one of the steroid hormones made in the adrenal gland-triangle-shaped organs at the top of your kidneys. Most cells within the body have cortisol receptors called the glucocorticoid receptor (GR, or GCR), also known as NR3C1. We have this receptor in the abdominal about four times more than other parts of the body; that's why we can store fat in this area. 28 Secretion is controlled by the hypothalamus, the pituitary gland, and the adrenal gland, a combination of glands often related to the HPA axis. Cortisol can help regulate blood sugar levels, regulate metabolism, help reduce inflammation, support memory formulation, control your sleep and wake cycle, and boost energy so you can handle stress and restore balance afterward. It has a controlling effect on salt and water balance and helps control blood pressure. You don't want it too much or too little; you want it just the right amount.

Let's see the picture. Once you have stress coming into your body, just protect yourself by releasing the cortisol. Cortisol is not evil; however, nowadays, we have more stress, our body tries to help us by releasing cortisol, but our body does not know the stress is coming from the tiger or it's coming from a traffic jam or just a simple email that causes stress to you. It's your natural "fight to fight" response that has saved our ancestors alive while they ran away from the tiger or helped humans survive most times. So, what can you do about it?

1. No stress. It will resolve all cortisol problems if you manage your stress. Therefore, practicing meditation and mindfulness is extremely helpful in controlling your stress level.

2. Once you have stress, do something physical instead of eating. Remember, we have more cortisol receptors in our abdominal area, so stress eating is the worst thing to do because you store more fat. Why don't you use this opportunity to lift weight and

build muscles? You have more cortisol during stress, which means you can lift more than usual. If you can't go to the gym right when you have stress, do some push-ups, squats, plyometrics in place, so you get your HIIT in no time.

I'm a human, and I have stress as you do. I know it's hard to live with no stress. Too much cortisol can cause a condition called Cushing's syndrome. It can lead to rapid weight gain, skin bruises easily, muscle weakness, diabetes, high blood pressure, fatigue, impaired brain function, and many other health problems.

Most of the time, you aren't aware that you have stress. Every time the sympathetic nervous system is activated, you have stress.

There are 3 main types of stress put on your body daily

1. Physical stress

There can be significant injuries (macro-traumas) like slip and fall, car accidents that cause severe damage to the body. A minor event that causes injury (Micro-traumas) includes poor posture, sitting for long periods, repetitive motions, improper movements, and things we do daily.

2. Chemical stress

is in our environment, and sometimes it's hard to avoid. For example, the foods you eat, the cleaners you use, and the air you breathe contain chemicals. Some of this is beyond your control. Sometimes, it creates toxins in our bodies, causing infection, allergy, and food poisoning.

3. Emotional stress

is the most common stress you deal with daily. It can be something you don't like, then you have fear, anger, frustration, worry, and so on, or it can be a loss of a loved one or pet. You deal with money, work, relationships, family, and many things daily that lead to specific emotions.

The key to managing stress is your brain, your frontal lobes. The stress response is a lifesaver. It's normal for your body to react to something that threatens you in a critical situation. React to protect yourself. The stress response is necessary for lifesaving. The frontal lobes can determine when it's time to turn it off. If the frontal lobes don't work very well, then the stress response will work on the opposition and go on much longer and more robust than it is supposed to. That's why different people have different stress levels, and then they act differently. Some people can be calm, but others can freak out. So, it depends on how well the frontal lobes are working. The frontal lobes are like a light switch that can turn things off. 29

THE SECOND KEY. STOP STORING FAT.

How to create the solution and control stress.

1. Create a pattern interrupt. The reason that you have to stress is that the brain gets stuck in the habits. What we want to do is interrupt the pattern.

2. Nutrients can give the brain the nutrient to help it function better. I got you covered on this part. You will learn more in the next chapter.

3. Brain stimulation

4. Lifestyle modifications that affect hormones and neurotransmitters such as dopamine and serotonin booster, which I will share with you in the next chapter.

Solution

1. Aerobic exercise. It's a perfect thing to do because its pattern interrupts. It will get you away from the things that make you stressed, and it also stimulates the brain from movement and increases the oxygen to the brain. You can also reduce insulin during aerobic exercise.

2. HIIT (High-intensity interval training) Even though this type of exercise stimulates cortisol, the trick you can do in just a short period and create the growth hormone that opposes cortisol. By doing 15-30 seconds of HIIT and maxing out your heart rate, your body produces growth hormone much more than cortisol.

3. Yoga, it's a fantastic activity. It's a pattern interrupt and its brain stimulation. When you do it, you teach your brain to learn

different things. Yoga is a great activity to boost your brain's neurotransmitters. You can choose any kind of yoga but don't get into an upbeat and intense one because that increase cortisol.

4. Recovery. More doesn't mean it's better. Remember, we break muscle in the gym, but we build muscle by replenishing our body after. Rest and recovery are essential.

5. Breathing exercise, it's powerful because the sympathetic (the fight-or-flight response) and parasympathetic nervous system (the rest and digest or feed and breed responses) are tight to your breath. When you breathe in, that is sympathetic activity and when you breathe out is parasympathetic activity. You can balance it out by breathing in and breathing out. You try to control the slow breath out a little longer than slow breathing in.

6. Meditation. It's like breathing, but meditation is more about paying attention to your mind and changing your focus. It increases frontal lobes activity and its brain stimulation. It's about finding a profound place of peace, and the more you do it, you get a deeper level of relaxation. You get more and more pattern interrupt and brain stimulation.

7. Mindfulness, start looking on the bright side. Mindfulness is the ability to be present, aware of what you are doing and where you are, and not reactive or overwhelmed by what is going on around you. It might go along with meditation, but mindfulness is deeper than meditation. You bring the practice with you all day long.

> Love Life Live Aloha!
>
> (My motto)
>
> Aloha (/əˈloʊhɑː/, Hawaiian: [əˈlohə]) is the Hawaiian word for love, affection, peace, compassion, and mercy, that is commonly used as a simple greeting. But has a more profound cultural and spiritual significance to native Hawaiians. The term is used to define a force that holds together an existence. 30

8. Gratitude is a warm feeling of thankfulness for the beautiful world we live in. It's an acknowledgment of the goodness in your life. It helps you to feel more positive emotions.

9. Celebrate and appreciate. When something good happens or a meaningful day like a birthday or anniversary. You should take time out for a bit of fun and self-congratulations. Enjoy the beautiful things in life and know that you deserve it. You can do it without food rewards involved. Here are some fun ideas; take a break, either a staycation or a vacation, write a gratitude letter to yourself, gather with friends and family, give yourself extra time for your favorite activities, it's a little thing count, for example, an additional time at your favorite coffee shop or, buy yourself some flowers.

10. Read a book or listen to audiobooks. It's a pattern interruption when you take your mind out of something and read or learn something new. Reading is a way to escape your world, and it can bring you to another world. Reading also stimulates your brain and imagination and keeps your brain healthy.

11. Listen to music and dance or sing out loud. I love doing this. Once my body moves, everything flows. Singing is a pattern interruption as well. You will focus on the words and rhythms.

12. Watching a movie. Yes, it will bring you to another world, and it's a pattern interruption.

13. Being with positive people and avoiding negative people. When you surround yourself with a positive influence, it will create positive energy throughout your day. It will be much easier to accomplish anything in your life.

14. The essential oil can create a pattern interrupt. When you inhale, the scent molecules in essential oil travel from the olfactory nerves to the brain, especially the amygdala, which plays a vital role in processing memory, decision-making, and emotional responses. I have practiced aromatherapy for over 20 years. I can give you some quick tips.

For boosting energy level, focus, and mood. Eucalyptus helps to stimulate the brain and improve energy. You can choose peppermint, citrus, i.e., wild orange, lime, lemon, grapefruit, rosemary, and spearmint is also suitable for increasing focus. I can write about the essential oil for another entire book.

15. Herbs like adaptogen that can calm you down; ashwagandha, kava, Siberian ginseng, Rhodiola, licorice root, Schisandra berry, tulsi, or holy basil, turmeric, cordyceps, maca, alma berry, astragalus root, and Gotu Kola.

Bacopa monnieri (Brahmi)

Give "Brahmi" a blessing herb a try. Brahmi is a staple plant in traditional Ayurvedic medicine is not only contain a powerful antioxidant but also helps reduce stress and anxiety by elevating your mood and reducing levels of cortisol, from research on an effective anti-stress agent (adaptogen) from plants found an extract of Bacopa monniera against acute (AS) and chronic stress (CS) models in rats. The study shows it may boost brain function, reduce inflammation, help reduce ADHD symptoms, help lower blood pressure levels, and have anti-cancer properties. [31] [32] [33] [34] [35] [36]

16. Smile and laugh.

> *A good laugh heals a lot of hurts- Madeleine L'Engle.*

Smiling can trick your brain into happiness. Research at the University of Kansas found that smiling helps reduce the body's response to stress and lower heart rate intense situations.

17. Sleep increases growth hormones, especially between 10:00 pm. - 2:00 am. It's important to get sleep for recovery.

18. Vitamin D3 and vitamin B1 and B5 help support the brain and the adrenal gland. You don't want to get vitamin B1 and B5 from supplements; you want to get it from food. The best source is nutritional yeast.

19. Spending time with your dog. Studies showed dogs could boost oxytocin hormones. (The love hormone) [37]

In Conclusion

Now you understand your hormones related to storing fat, and you know how to deal with it. Next chapter, I will dive deep into overcoming sugar and refined carb cravings and addiction.

TO-DO LIST:

Write at least 5 stress relievers you like on your notebook or paper.

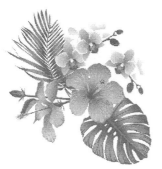

CHAPTER 4

OVERCOME SUGAR, REFINED CARB CRAVINGS, AND SUGAR ADDICTION WITH SCIENCE-BASED STRATEGIES

IS SUGAR ADDICTION REAL?

According to the research on the biochemical and neurobehavioral consequences of sugar consumption has been found to produce more symptoms than is required to be considered an addictive substance. Animal data have shown a significant overlap between the consumption of added sugars and drug-like effects, including bingeing, craving, tolerance, withdrawal, cross-sensitization, cross-tolerance, cross-dependence, reward, and opioid effects. Sugar addiction depends on the natural endogenous opioids released upon sugar intake. In both animals and humans, the evidence in the literature shows substantial parallels and overlap between drugs of abuse and sugar from the standpoint of brain neurochemistry and behavior. [38] [39]

WHAT IS SUGAR ADDICTION?

Do you have a sugar addiction? Someone's answers may be a little addicting. Well, if you are sugar-addicted, you are addicted. It's not a little or more. For example, you can't say you are a little pregnant. If you are pregnant, you are pregnant, not a little pregnant or more pregnant.

My clients and some of my friends asked me. Can you please help me? I'm eating to death. I know I shouldn't eat this food.

Am I crazy? Why am I doing this?

Why am I not normal and act like a bad person? I can't control myself!

I'm a sugar addict, and I'm a refined carbohydrate addict.

I can't stop drinking! What's wrong with me?

During my transition going through a divorce in my late 30 and early 40, I became addicted to refined carbohydrates like chips and cookies, and I couldn't stop drinking wine. Once I drink, I will go through the entire bottle by myself. I relied on exercise because I know how to burn calories correctly and efficiently since I've been a certified personal trainer for over 15 years. My fasting blood glucose was high, and my hemoglobin A1c level was high. I couldn't believe it once I saw my blood test result. I ate healthy, many vegetables, fruits, and whole foods. But my problem was I couldn't stop eating refined carbohydrates and drinking. The doctor described my condition as a prediabetic from my blood test result, which shocked me and made me cry and hurt so deeply. How can someone like me, healthy and fit, have a prediabetic?

I just understood what was going on with me a few years ago. At the end-of-year 2017, I had an accident and slipped and fell. Since then, I couldn't move much, and of course, I couldn't exercise. But I had more time to read. Thank you, God. Thank you for what's happening to me. My eyes were open, and I had the answer for my health, and I'm going to share it with you. Since I moved to Hawaii, I also did several detoxes, but the one was incredible and stopped me from addiction. It's during lent in March 2019. It might be another book that I will write about soon. In this book, I want to share with you a science-based strategy.

Since I got into an accident, I had more time to slow down and read many books. I usually read nutrition, anti-aging, and beauty books through food and natural sources. However, I came across the research related to the subject and went through brain chemistry.

Sugar addiction is real. It's not something in your imagination. Your brain is brilliant, and it's more intelligent than you. It's not your fault that you are addicted to sugar or refined carbohydrates. Sugar has a property changing your brain chemistry quickly. We will often see a mixture of fat & sugar (including refined carbs) together, such as donuts, chips, pastries, ice cream, or fast food.

I want to explain what happens in the brain when someone has an addiction to carbs. A little center called "Nucleus"- a tiny cell body called the nucleus accumbens. It's deep in the brain. [8] It's way deep inside, right in the center. It is a nucleus, a part of the body's reward systems that uses dopamine as its primary neurotransmitter and GABA and serotonin. These neurotransmitters are intimately involved in creating this pleasure sensation. Certain recreational drugs, alcohol, exercise, tobacco, sex, and sugar will return to this center when this nucleus is stimulated. This little trigger causes a little cell body to release these neurotransmitters to give you the sensation of pleasure. It does not give the sensation directly. They do it indirectly through the nucleus. You feel this because of your body chemistry.

---

[8] Avena, N. M., Rada, P., & Hoebel, B. G. (2008). Evidence for sugar addiction: behavioral and neurochemical effects of intermittent, excessive sugar intake. Neuroscience and biobehavioral reviews, 32(1), 20–39. https://doi.org/10.1016/j.neubiorev.2007.04.019

On an MRI, when people take sugar, the center lights up like a laser. So, it's up. It's involved in all the release of dopamine and pleasure. [9] People get pleasure by consuming refined carbohydrates because refined carbohydrates quickly turn into sugar. The problem is too much of this. The stimulus downgrades the receptor for dopamine, and now you're not satisfied, so you need a little more in a little more until, eventually, you create an addiction. [10]

Unlike many other substances use disorders or behavioral compulsions, sugar addiction, is often easy to spot. The most unmistakable signs of sugar addiction involve consuming large amounts of food or drinks laden with sugar. The individual may eat constantly, combat boredom, and become hyper and crash. They may even talk about craving sugar after stressful life experiences. We can see the sugar addiction with emotional eating, binge eating, anxiety, and alcoholism.

IT IS NOT YOUR FAULT. IT'S YOUR BRAIN.

So, no worries. I have you covered with the plan. You will know how to handle them and overcome your sugar and refined carbs addiction.

Overcome sugar addiction by understanding neurotransmitters.

---

[9] Fowler, J. S., Volkow, N. D., Kassed, C. A., & Chang, L. (2007). Imaging the addicted human brain. Science & practice perspectives, 3(2), 4–16. https://doi.org/10.1151/spp07324

[10] Substance Abuse and Mental Health Services Administration (US); Office of the Surgeon General (US). Facing Addiction in America: The Surgeon General's Report on Alcohol, Drugs, and Health [Internet]. Washington (DC): US Department of Health and Human Services;

2016 Nov. CHAPTER 2, THE NEUROBIOLOGY OF SUBSTANCE USE, MISUSE, AND ADDICTION. Available from: https://www.ncbi.nlm.nih.gov/books/NBK424849/

Dopamine and serotonin are both neurotransmitters. Neurotransmitters are chemical messengers used by the nervous system that regulate countless functions and processes in your body, from sleep to metabolism.

Serotonin.

What is serotonin?

Serotonin is an important brain chemical. Serotonin promotes relaxation, calm, peace, positivity, and satiety.

Low serotonin may be linked with mood issues, seasonal affective disorder (SAD), premenstrual syndrome (PMS), menopause symptoms, chronic alcohol use, or insulin resistance. Any of these can cause sugar cravings. Serotonin plays an essential role in regulating sleep and mood, and women have lower serotonin issues when compared to men, who mostly have lower dopamine levels.

Attention!!! Ladies.

As premenstrual serotonin drops, PMS may occur. PMS includes many discomforts: anxiety, irritability, mood swings, nervousness, angry outbursts, impulsivity, fatigue, fluid retention, bloating, weight gain, backache, headaches, joint pain, breast pain, acne, increased appetite, insomnia, and cravings, especially for sugar. Women with PMS consume more sugar, alcohol, refined carbohydrate, salty food, fatty food, caffeine, and dairy products.

Sugar also increases the intensity of PMS symptoms. [41]

So, when diagnosed with depression. Serotonin meds are given to boost their serotonin levels. They are getting better and feel more optimistic about life and the future. They have more self-esteem and confidence. However, taking medications that increase serotonin leads to side effects- "Serotonin syndrome" can occur. Too much serotonin can cause mild symptoms such as shivering, heavy sweating, confusion, restlessness, headaches, high blood pressure, twitching muscles, and diarrhea. More severe symptoms include high fever, unconsciousness, seizures, or irregular heartbeat.

SET YOURSELF UP FOR SUCCESS.

After learning what serotonin is and what's the trigger? Now, are you ready to learn more tips and create a good mood hormone?

How to increase serotonin naturally

1. Adding serotonin-boosting foods to your diet.

Your brain needs amino acid tryptophan and folate, vitamin B6, vitamin C, zinc, and magnesium to create serotonin.

Important factor: Your body converts tryptophan in your diet into the 5-HTP, which is then converted into serotonin. However, your body can't just convert without specific vitamins and minerals needed to activate the chemical process. Therefore, keep in mind that you need to eat folate, vitamin B6, vitamin C, zinc, and magnesium for optimal serotonin production.

If you do not get enough vitamins and minerals, you might also have trouble sleeping. Why does that happen? It's because serotonin metabolizes into melatonin. If you do not have a sufficient sleep, you may crave sugar and junk foods the following day.

To get the maximum benefit of the serotonin-boosting trick, you will need to eat seven servings of vegetables and fruits every day to ensure that you will get the vitamins and minerals that support serotonin production.

High tryptophan foods include chicken, turkey, red meat, pork, tofu, fish, beans, milk, nuts, seeds, oatmeal, and eggs. The recommended daily intake for tryptophan is 4mg per kilogram of body weight or 1.8mg per pound. Therefore, a person weighing 70kg (~154 pounds) should consume around 280mg of tryptophan per day.

Below is a list of the **top 10 foods highest in tryptophan** calculated for someone weighing 70kg (154lbs). [42]

Table 1: Top 10 food highest in Tryptophan

Food	Amount	Tryptophan mg.
1. Lean chicken or turkey	6 oz.	687 mg
2. Beef (skirt steak)	6 oz.	636 mg
3. Lean pork chop	6 oz.	627 mg
4. Firm tofu	1 cup	592 mg
5. Fish (salmon)	6 oz.	570 mg
6. Boil soybeans (Edamame)	1 cup	416 mg
7. Milk	16 oz glass	211 mg
8. Squash and pumpkin seeds	1 oz.	164 mg
9. Oatmeal	1 cup	94 mg
10. Eggs	1 large	77 mg

More Poultry High in Tryptophan

Ground turkey, roast chicken, turkey breast, roast duck, turkey drumstick, and a chicken leg. (drumstick)

More Lean Red Meat High in Tryptophan

Roast lamb, beef stew (chuck), buffalo sirloin steak, and hamburger patty. (97% lean)

More Pork Products High in Tryptophan

Roast ham, rack of pork ribs, roast boar, and bratwurst sausage.

More Soy Foods High in Tryptophan

Soy milk, sprouted soybeans, and tempeh.

More Fish High in Tryptophan

Tuna, cod, tilapia, and Mahi Mahi.

More Cooked Legumes High in Tryptophan

White beans, red kidney beans, pinto beans, black beans, and lentils.

More Dairy Products High in Tryptophan

Cottage Cheese, hard mozzarella, cheddar cheese, parmesan, gruyere, and yogurt.

More Nuts and Seeds High in Tryptophan

Chia seeds, flax seeds, pistachios, and peanuts.

More Cooked Whole Grains High in Tryptophan

Teff, quinoa, and brown rice.

Table 2: Top 10 food highest in B6

The daily value (% DV) for vitamin B6 is 1.7mg per day

Food	Amount	B6 mg.
1. Salmon	6 oz.	1.6 mg
2. Lean chicken breast	6 oz.	1.6 mg
3. Fortified tofu	1 cup	1.1 mg
4. Lean pork chop	6 oz.	0.9 mg
5. Beef (skirt steak)	6 oz.	0.8 mg
6. Sweet potato	1 cup mash	0.6 mg
7. Banana	1 cup sliced	0.6 mg
8. Potatoes	A medium	0.5 mg
9. Avocado	1 fruit	0.5 mg
10. Pistachio nut	1 oz.	0.5 mg

Table 3: Top 10 food highest in folate

The current daily value (% DV) for folate (Vitamin B9) is 400 µg

Food	Amount	Folate
1. Edamame	1 cup	482 µg
2. Lentil	1 cup	358 µg
3. Asparagus	1 cup cooked	268 µg
4. Spinach	1 cup cooked	263 µg
5. Broccoli	1 cup cooked	168 µg
6. Avocado	Per fruit	163 µg
7. Mango	1 cup	71 µg
8. Lettuce	1 cup	64 µg
9. Sweet corn	1 cup cooked	61 µg
10. Orange	1 cup	482 µg

Table 4: Top 10 foods highest in Vitamin C, ranked by common serving size. The current daily value (% DV) for vitamin C is 90 mg.

Food	Amount	Vitamin C mg.
1. Guavas	1 cup	377 mg
2. Kiwi	1 cup	167 mg
3. Sweet bell peppers	1 cup	152 mg
4. Strawberries	1 cup	98 mg
5. Oranges	1 cup	96 mg
6. Papaya	1 cup	88 mg
7. Broccoli	1 cup	81 mg
8. Tomato	1 cup cooked	55 mg
9. Snow peas	1 cup	38 mg
10. Kale	1 cup cooked	23 mg

Table 5: Top 10 foods highest in zinc, ranked by common serving size.

The current daily value (DV) for Zinc is 11mg.

Food	Amount	Zinc mg.
1. Oyster	6 oysters	52 mg
2. Beef (chuck steak)	5 oz.	15 mg
3. Chicken legs	Per leg	5 mg
4. Firm Tofu	1 cup	4 mg
5. Lean pork chop	6 oz.	4 mg
6. Hemp seeds	1 oz.	3 mg
7. Lentil	1 cup	3 mg
8. Yogurt	1 cup	2 mg
9. Oatmeal	1 cup	2 mg
10. Shiitake mushroom	1 cup cooked	2 mg

Table 6: Top 10 foods highest in magnesium ranked by common serving size. The current daily value (DV) for magnesium is 420mg.

Food	Amount	Magnesium mg.
1. Spinach	1 cup cooked	157 mg
2. Squash or pumpkin seeds	1 oz.	156 mg
3. Lima beans	1 cup cooked	126 mg
4. Tuna	6 oz.	109 mg
5. Brown rice	1 cup	86 mg
6. Almonds	1 oz.	77 mg
7. Dark chocolate (85% cacao)	1 oz.	65 mg
8. Avocado	Per fruit	58 mg
9. Yogurt	1 cup	47 mg
10. Bananas	1 cup sliced	41 mg

The best way to do it is to have low glycemic index carbs with your protein and vegetables. For example,

Salmon (Tryptophan & B6), broccoli (folate) + Kale (Vitamin C), shiitake mushroom (Zinc), brown rice (Magnesium)

Now you got Tryptophan ---> 5-HTP ---> Serotonin

2. **Adding serotonin-boosting activities.**

During the 21 days of sugar detox, you will also add boosting activities to your daily routine. Feeling anxious and fearful is a sign that you are low in serotonin. Just add a little each day, and you will see incredible results. [43]

My favorite top 10 serotonin-boosting activities.

1. Walking along the beach in the evening and watching the sunset.
2. Listening to my favorite music.
3. Dancing while listening to the music.
4. Walking and playing with my dog.
5. Cooking yummy food.
6. Swimming and getting some sunshine.
7. Reading books and studies about nutrition and health.
8. Breathing with essential oils.
9. Giving myself a face mask or scrubs.
10. Getting a massage.

Remember in chapter 2, one of the to-do lists is "smile," that's serotonin-boosting activities as well.

Do you need more ideas?

- Something makes you happy, such as flowers, pictures, children, animals, or anything that you see and brightens up your day.

- Some lovely activities include holding hands, kissing, making love, calling just to say, "I love you," hugging, and giving or getting a massage.

- Doing something for someone, such as volunteering, opening the door for someone, complimenting someone, or sending a card to friends or family.

- Sport or outdoor activities include walking, jogging, fishing, beach volleyball, swimming, Kayaking, or horseback riding.

3. **Say hello to SUNSHINE.**

Research shows that your brain makes more of the feel-good neurotransmitter serotonin on sunny days than it does on darker days. [44]

Sunlight and darkness trigger the release of hormones in your brain. Welcoming the sunshine in the morning after waking up is most beneficial, typically within the first hour of crawling out of bed.

Sunlight increases the brain's release of serotonin hormone, which boosts mood and helps you feel calm and focused. At night, darker lighting triggers the brain to make another melatonin hormone. This hormone helps you sleep.

From the research, when people are exposed to sunlight or very bright artificial light in the morning, their nocturnal melatonin production occurs sooner, and they enter into sleep more easily at night. Melatonin production also shows a seasonal variation relative to light availability, with the hormone produced for a more extended period in the winter than in the summer. The melatonin rhythm phase advancement caused by exposure to bright morning light effectively against insomnia, premenstrual syndrome, and seasonal affective disorder (SAD). [45]

If you want to get the benefit of morning sunlight therapy, going shade-free in the daylight, even for just 10–15 minutes, could confer significant health benefits—sunlight cues particular areas in the retina, which triggers the release of serotonin. However, if you want to get vitamin D, aim for at least 30 minutes. From the study, for most white people, a half-hour in the summer sun in a bathing suit can start the release of 50,000 IU (1.25 mg) vitamin D into the circulation within 24 hours of exposure; this same amount of exposure yields 20,000–30,000 IU in tanned individuals and 8,000–10,000 IU in dark-skinned people.

My best advice for sunshine therapy is walking outside 30-45 minutes in the morning without sunglasses or visors and letting your retina soak the sun. It's ok to apply sunscreen on your face.

I like to go swimming in the morning during the summer to get the sunlight through my skin & eyes and my daily exercise. However, it's too cold in wintertime (between December - February), yes, I live in Hawaii, and we don't have wintertime. Anyway, it is too cold for me to swim before 10:00 am during those months. Walking is perfect for everyone to boost vitamin D and serotonin hormones. However, if you don't have time for walking in the morning.

Here are my tips.

1. Sit outside early in the morning during your morning beverage, either a cup of tea or coffee. Whether you have a balcony or backyard, both are great, as long as you get your sunshine.

2. Stretch or do morning yoga 30 minutes or longer in the sun once you get up at your own home and do it outdoors.

3. If you have a garden, do your activities with your plants in the morning. They will love it, and so do you.

4. Walk your dog in the morning.

5. Walk your children to school.

6. Drive with no sunglasses in the morning.

7. Keep your eyes outside the window. If you have to be in the office or building during the day,

4. **Boosting serotonin with meditation.**

Many studies have shown that meditation can increase serotonin levels and melatonin, which helps you sleep. [46] In addition, studies show that the rhythmic stimulation of music promotes the release of endorphins, dopamine, and serotonin, affecting brain chemistry and resulting in stress reduction and mood elevation. The serotonin booster uses Alpha frequencies at 10 Hertz, a known mood-elevating frequency associated with the release of serotonin. [47]

The alpha frequencies are used to promote a calming effect that will entertain your brain to a relaxed but "in the flow" state, not one that will make you feel sleepy.

5. **Exercise increases tryptophan.**

In many studies, exercise has been shown to increase serotonin production and release. Especially aerobic exercises, like running, walking, and cycling, are the most likely to boost serotonin.[48.]

If you can exercise outdoors, it's better than indoors. Apart from that, you can burn more calories. You can also get vitamin D and help you sleep better too. Make exercise an essential part of your routine, even though you don't feel you want to do it, but after 15 minutes of movement, you will feel much better, and you can even go for a longer session.

Here is a fun idea for you.

- Stress # goes for a bike ride.

- Angry # Try kickboxing.

- Rushed # try HIIT.

- Anxious # goes for a walk.

- Lonely # try a group class.

- Feeling stuck # going for a run or walking.

- Worried # Try yoga.

- Sad # turn on the music and dance.

- Altogether, # go to the beach.

My mantra B.E.A.C.H.

Best escape anyone can have.

Best enjoyment anyone can have.

6. Positive thought & positive affirmation.

Positive affirmation is a powerful tool for self-transformation. Most of the time, low serotonin levels produce anxiety and fear. Under any circumstances, anxiety and other forms of stress deplete your serotonin.

Does the problem start with stress or lower serotonin?

No doctor can answer those questions for you, and it doesn't matter. Once you start on that downward circle, you will keep going unless you intentionally break the cycle. You need to either change your thoughts or boost serotonin levels- or both.

Your thoughts are powerful, affecting your mood and your physical body. Once you identify the negative statement that you think about yourself, change it to a positive one. I love to listen to audiobooks that help me transform my negative thoughts of myself or situations into a positive one.

The key to this is understanding your negative thoughts. Every thought we think is creating our future.

If you thought that reflects anxiety, worry, negative and a lack of confidence.

- Something terrible is going to happen to me.

- If I'm not successful today, I'm a failure.

- He might think I'm selfish if I don't do this.

- They think I'm fat.

- I'm not good enough, that's why my boyfriend left me.

Do anything of this sound familiar? If one of these sentences describes how you think about yourself and your surroundings. Now we have found the negative thought and pattern. But if they didn't match your thoughts, let's write about what is negative, though then we can get to the start point. Okay! Right down to at least 5 sentences now.

Ready? Let's transform your thoughts. Then you will be transferred to a new you who is happy and lovable. If you always think, "I'm not good enough. Let's change that. First, you don't need to be perfect. The perfect life does not exist. So that's why we come to learn about life on earth. Stop getting stuck in the comparison trap and social media. What is good for them might not be suitable for you. So, when this negative thought arises.

- Write in your notebook.

- Then write at least 5 beautiful memories you have.

- Get back to those negative thoughts and identify the trigger and change that. For example, when you are upset with your belly fat, you compare yourself to other slim ladies and have no belly fat.

I would write about that trigger instead of being upset. You would use that tool to be your motivation. Most of the time, if someone is looking fabulous, I'm sure they pay attention to the little detail of their body. They are feeding their body with good, healthy food, and they spend time exercising and pampering themselves. If they can do it for a reasonable amount of time, you can do it too. So set up your goals and change the habit. What do you need to look fabulous?

1. Feeding yourself with good, nourishing food. If you don't know what good nourish food is, find a helper. Right now, you are reading my book, and that's a positive sign you will learn. Knowledge is wisdom. Once you know it, then you apply it to your life.

2. Spending your time in the kitchen and preparing a good meal.

3. Exercise. How much time can you put in? Write it down if you don't know how to and where to start. If there is a will, there is a way. There's a lot of information out there for you to learn. Please join the Facebook community to learn from me and others.

4. Pamper yourself. If you love something, you should take care of it. You are in this body in this lifetime, so make it your temple. Take care of it. In the 21 days sugar detox program, I also include a pamper party to take care of your body from the inside out.

I can tell you that beautiful things will happen if you spend time and focus on it. Every time I teach yoga, I tell my students to go at their own pace. Do not compare the level of flexibility of other students with themself or me.

Why is that? First, I have practiced yoga since I was 18 years old, so it's been over 20 years. Therefore, if you just start, you can't compare with someone who has been doing it for a long time. Second, I love yoga. I do it regularly for this reason. I have more hours of practicing yoga. It's like a weight loss journey. Someone who looks fabulous. She has been eating clean for a long time. It's not a diet for her anymore, but a lifestyle. If you just started this year, you know that you just started. It's like driving. You want to go cross-country from Stanford, Connecticut, to San Francisco, California. It's 2,939 miles, and it will take 43 hours and 10 minutes without stopping. However, if you want to stop and sleep at the hotel, it's ok so long as you keep driving. Look at this scenario.

1. Car number 1 keeps moving, stops to sleep, and stops in every state. It will take longer, but it will get to the destination.

2. Car number 2 starts and stops in Utah for a few months, so car number 2 will get to San Francisco a few months after car number 1.

3. Car number 3 starts simultaneously and does not want to stop because they have few people to take a turn to drive, so they get to the destination faster than car number 1 and 2.

4. Car number 4 wants to get to San Francisco too, but they didn't leave Connecticut because they didn't set up the date to leave, they didn't have a plan, they kept postponing the date. So, car number 4 won't get to San Francisco because they didn't take action.

This example it's like weight loss. You will need to take action and keep going. It will take longer to get to your destiny if you keep stopping.

Whatever you do with your journey, enjoy it and do it with love, and spice it with fun.

Another pitfall, if deep down your thought is" I'm not safe," I want to give you a guide to change it to be a more optimistic message, such as "All is well" or "Things will turn out okay"

I love my morning affirmation, and I have been doing it for a few years now. I can tell you it has had a significant impact on my life. You can check out my other book, <u>Daily Affirmations for Prosperity and Happiness: 500 Positive Affirmations to Reset Your Brain.</u> I am sure it will transform your thoughts on the bright side.

"You are not a helpless victim of your own thoughts, but rather a master of your own mind." Louise Hay.

7. **Supplement.**

If all-natural serotonin booster tips don't work for you or are in a stressful situation, you can try the supplement to boost the serotonin. Many studies have shown that supplements can treat serotonin deficiencies like 5-HTP, St. John's Wort, green tea, and turmeric. [49]

UNLOCK THE SECOND SECRET

Dopamine.

What is dopamine?

Dopamine is a neurotransmitter released by the brain that plays several roles in humans and other animals. Some of its special functions are in [50]

- movements

- memory

- pleasurable reward

- behavior, and cognition

- attention

- inhibition of prolactin production

- sleep

- mood

- learning

Dopamine plays a role in how we feel pleasure. It's a big part of our uniquely human ability to think and plan. It helps us strive, focus, and find things interesting. This means food, sex, and several drugs of abuse are also stimulants of dopamine release in the brain, in areas such as the nucleus accumbens and prefrontal cortex. This brain chemical is associated with challenges and thrills, such as watching exciting sports matches, racing a car, driving fast, or even the pushing chemical that you seek love and sex. When dopamine is at a healthy level, life is fun and exciting, but once you lack dopamine, it can make you unmotivated, bored, sad, have a low sex drive, have a short attention span, have a low work performance, isolate yourself, emotional eating, and you can't focus on your goals. Low dopamine levels can bring us rushing for a quick-fix food, drugs, and behaviors. Foods with bad fat send our brains to release a temporary amount of dopamine, giving us a feeling of rush, excitement, and pleasure. So, we keep eating those foods for a quick fix while shrinking our brains.

Several conditions and stimuli cause low dopamine. The most common causes related to Low Dopamine levels are.

- Stress

- Alcohol Withdrawal Syndrome

- Obesity

- Unhealthy nutrition

- Parkinson's Disease

- Restless leg syndrome disorder, and creativity; One of the most unfathomable causes of dopamine deficiency is high creativity. Highly creative people often suffer from low dopamine levels in their brains. Although they produce high dopamine levels, they lack dopamine D2 receptors in their thalamus. I also fall for this one. Big time!

- Use of drugs

- Other factors responsible for dopamine levels to decrease is lack of sleep, hypothyroidism, exposure to lead, arsenic, and cadmium, tyrosine deficiency, deficiency of magnesium, zinc, iron and vitamin B3, B6, C, and D, Insufficient adrenals, estrogen, the inefficiency of Human growth hormone. [51]

Dopamine deficiency is the result- and craving fat, caffeine, and sometimes sugar, which combine with fat. Low dopamine can lead to depression, emotional eating, and binge eating.

So, what can we do about that? Here I got your answer.

HOW TO WIN THE GAME

Increase dopamine a healthy way.

1. **Eating food to increase dopamine.**

First, let's get to know dopamine a little more. Dopamine can be made from the amino acid tyrosine, found in many foods, such as beef, pork, fish, chicken, tofu, milk, cheese, beans, seeds, nuts, and whole grains.

Your body converts tyrosine from the food you eat into L-DOPA and then dopamine.

However, your body can't process this chemical efficiently without specific vitamins and minerals. Those vitamins and minerals are vitamin C, iron, folate, and copper.

The recommended daily tyrosine intake is 25mg per kilogram of body weight or 11 mg per pound. A person weighing 70kg (~154 pounds) should consume around 875mg of tyrosine per day, which is used to calculate the recommended daily intake. [52]

Table 7: Top 10 foods highest in tyrosine

Food	Amount	Tyrosine mg.
1. Beef (Skirt steak)	6 oz.	2174 mg
2. Lean pork chop	6 oz.	2088 mg
3. Fish (Salmon)	6 oz.	2052 mg
4. Lean chicken breast	6 oz.	1964 mg
5. Firm tofu	1 cup	1767 mg
6. Milk	16 oz.	833 mg
7. Low-fat ricotta cheese	½ cup	739 mg
8. Large white bean	1 cup	490 mg
9. Squash and pumpkin seeds	1 oz.	306 mg
10. Wild rice	1 cup	277 mg

ranked by common serving size. 875 mg. = 100% of the recommended

daily intake (%RDI) for a 70kg person (~154 pounds)

More Red Meat High in Tyrosine, such as lamb roast, beef stew, beef chuck roast, buffalo steak, and beef hamburger.

More Pork Products High in Tyrosine, such as roasted ham, broiled tenderloin, and spareribs.

Fish High in Tyrosine, such as tuna, grouper, snapper, tilapia fillet, and cod.

More Poultry High in Tyrosine, such as whole chicken leg, ground turkey, chicken breast (chopped), turkey breast, and a single chicken thigh

More Soy Foods High in tyrosine, such as tempeh (fermented tofu), boiled soybeans (edamame), natto, soybean sprouts and soy milk

More Dairy High in Tyrosine, such as nonfat yogurt, plain (whole fat) yogurt, and low-fat buttermilk

More Cheese High in Tyrosine, such as cottage cheese, parmesan cheese, Swiss cheese, provolone cheese, and gouda cheese.

More Beans and Lentils High in Tyrosine include lentils, split peas, red kidney beans, navy beans, and black beans.

More Nuts and Seeds are High in tyrosine, such as hemp seeds, peanuts, toasted sesame seeds, sunflower seeds, and chia seeds.

More Whole Grains High in Tyrosine, such as teff, oatmeal, Kamut, millet, whole-wheat pasta, and brown rice.

Table 8: Top 10 foods highest in iron

Ranked by typical serving size.[11] 18 g of iron= 100% of the daily value

Food	Amount	Iron mg.
1. Fortified cereal	¾ cup	19.6 mg
2. Beef (Skirt steak)	6 oz.	9.3 mg
3. Shellfish (oysters)	3 oz.	7.8 mg
4. Dried fruits (Apricot)	1 cup	7.5 mg
5. Large white bean	1 cup	6.6 mg
6. Spinach	1 cup cooked	6.4 mg
7. Baking chocolate (Unsweetened)	1 oz. Square	5 mg
8. Quinoa	1 cup	2.8 mg
9. White button mushrooms	1 cup	2.7 mg
10. Squash and pumpkin seeds	1 oz.	2.5 mg

More Red Meat High in Iron

- 28% DV in a 3oz slice of beef liver

- 16% DV in a 3oz buffalo steak

---

[11] Whitbread, D. (2021, July 28). Top 10 Foods Highest in Iron. My Food Data. https://www.myfooddata.com/articles/food-sources-of-iron.php

- 14% DV in a 3oz beef chuck roast

- 14% DV in a 3oz lean ground beef patty (burger)

- 13% DV in a 3oz lamb shoulder roast

- 11% DV per 3oz of beef short rib

More Seafood High in Iron (%DV per 3oz)

- 51% DV per 3oz of cuttlefish

- 48% DV per 3oz of whelk

- 45% DV per 3oz of octopus

- 32% DV per 3oz of mussels

- 18% DV per 3oz of abalone

- 14% DV per 3oz of scallops

More Dried Fruit High in Iron

- 36% DV per cup of dried peaches

- 26% DV per cup of dried prunes

- 17% DV per cup of dried figs

- 17% DV per cup of dried raisins

- 7% DV per cup of dried apples

More Beans High in Iron

- 49% DV per up of soybeans

- 37% DV per cup of lentils

- 29% DV per cup of kidney beans

- 26% DV per cup of garbanzo beans (chickpeas)

- 25% DV per cup of lima beans

- 24% DV per cup of navy beans

- 20% DV per cup of black beans

- 20% DV per cup of pinto beans

- 20% DV per cup of black-eyed peas

More Green Leafy Vegetables High in Iron

- 22% DV per cup of cooked Swiss chard

- 16% DV per cup of cooked turnip greens

- 15% DV per cup of cooked beet greens

- 14% DV per cup of cooked Scotch (curly) kale

- 14% DV per cup of raw mustard spinach

- 6% DV per cup of raw kale

- 5% DV per cup of raw beet greens

More Chocolate High in Iron

- 66% DV in 1 cup of cocoa powder

- 19% DV in 1oz of dark chocolate (70%-85% cocoa)

- 13% DV in 1oz of semi-dark chocolate (45%-59% cocoa)

- 6% DV per 1.5oz candy bar

- 6% DV per 1/2 cup of chocolate mousse

More Wholegrains High in Iron

- 12% DV per cup of oatmeal

- 12% DV per cup of barley

- 11% DV per cup of rice

- 10% DV per cup of bulgur

- 7% DV per cup of buckwheat

- 6% DV per cup of millet

More Mushrooms High in Iron

- 45% DV per cup of sliced morels

- 14% DV per cup of straw mushrooms

- 10% DV per cup of chanterelles

- 6% DV per cup of slices oyster mushrooms

- 4% DV per cup of sliced shiitake mushrooms

More Nuts & Seeds High in Iron

- 23% DV per oz of sesame seeds

- 13% DV per oz of hemp seeds

- 12% DV per oz of chia seeds

- 9% DV per oz of dry-roasted cashews

- 9% DV per oz of flax seeds

- 8% DV per oz of sunflower seeds

- 6% DV per oz of almonds

Table 9: Top 10 foods highest in copper

Ranked by common serving size. 0.9 mg of copper= 100% of the daily value [12]

Food	Amount	Copper mg.
1. Oysters	6 oysters	3.8 mg
2. Shiitake mushrooms	1 cup cooked	1.3 mg
3. Firm tofu	1 cup	1 mg
4. Sweet potato	1 cup mashed	0.7 mg
5. Sesame seeds	1 oz.	0.7 mg
6. Cashew	1 oz.	0.6 mg
7. Chickpea	1 cup	0.6 mg
8. Salmon	6 oz.	0.5 mg
9. Dark chocolate (70-85% cacao)	1 oz.	0.5 mg
10. Avocado	1 fruit	0.4 mg

So now you know why I mentioned the program with 7 servings of vegetables and fruits. Because it's so good for our brain.

2. Exercise helps to boost dopamine.

---

[12] Whitbread, D. (2021, July 28). Top 10 Foods Highest in Copper. My Food Data. https://www.myfooddata.com/articles/high-copper-foods.php

You might think she said it again and again about exercise because she is a personal trainer. No! It's not because of that. Physical exercise is one of the best things you can do for your brain. The research showed physical exercise increases the production of new brain cells, slows down brain cell aging, and increases dopamine levels. Exercise has also been associated with improved mood and overall, a better outlook on life. [53]

3. **Listen to music.**

Listening to calm music or natural sounds can increase pleasurable feelings, improve mood, reduce stress, and help with focus and concentration. Research has shown that much of this is achieved due to increased dopamine levels. [54] [55]

4. **Meditate.**

The complete health benefits of meditation have been shown through hundreds of research studies. Many have shown that meditation increases dopamine, improving concentration and focus. Suppose you have never meditated before. You can try a guided meditation for beginners. [56]

5. **Sleep**

To ensure that your brain increases dopamine, naturally, you will need to make sure that you get enough sleep. A mouse study suggests that sleep helps restore the brain by flushing out toxins that build up during waking hours. The results point to a potential new role in health and disease sleep. Lack of sleep has been shown to reduce concentrations of neurotransmitters, including dopamine and their receptors. [57]

6. **Get a massage.**

I'm sure everyone loves to get a massage. It can help to relax and get rid of stress. To keep dopamine levels high is to avoid stress, which is almost impossible these days. Research has shown that massage therapy activates neurotransmitters, increasing dopamine levels by 31% and serotonin by 28% while decreasing cortisol (a stress hormone) levels. [58]

7. **A positive affirmation.**

The negative thoughts in your head will ruin your attitude and reduce your dopamine level. I knew you didn't try to create it, but it just showed up in your head. It's better to learn how to transform a negative thought into a positive one.

<u>The negative one:</u> I never, ever succeeded.

<u>The positive one</u>

: I'm successful in being a wonderful person because I have been there for my family.

: I am incredibly successful because I have tried my best.

The negative one: My life is not going the way I want it to be.

The positive one: I have such a fantastic life, and I love my life.

The positive affirmation might not come naturally in the beginning. Once you have a positive thought, write it down and learn how to change it. You also can check out *my book; Daily Affirmation for Prosperity and Happiness; 500 Positive affirmations to reset your brain.*

8. **Supplement**

This is the last source. If you don't get better after trying the above 7 natural ways. You would need some supplements to boost your dopamine level.

1. <u>Amino acids</u> can help boost your dopamine level. There are three of them.

- L-Tyrosine

As I mentioned earlier, we can get L-Tyrosine from food but, if you can't get enough for any reason or if your body can't convert, especially during times of stress, exhaustion, or illness. You can take supplements instead of food sources.

- SAM-e (s-adenosylmethionine)

SAM-e is a normally existing compound in the body. While technically not an amino acid, it is a present metabolite of the amino acid l-methionine. SAM-e has been used in alternative medicine as a likely effective aid in reducing the symptoms of depression and in treating osteoarthritis. [59]

- L-Theanine

L-theanine is an amino acid found in green, black, and white teas. It enhances learning and promotes mood by increasing dopamine. It's one of the particular reasons you should include green tea in your daily diet because it can put you into a state of calm focus. If you prefer drinking tea to taking supplements, it's generally recommended you drink 3 cups of green tea per day for maximum benefits. [60] [61]

2. <u>Herbal remedies.</u>

- Mucuna Pruriens is a tropical legume, and the beans and pods contain L-dopa, a dopamine precursor. Mucuna supplements are sold to enhance mood, memory, overall brain health, anti-aging, and libido. [62]

- Ginkgo (Ginkgo biloba) is one of the oldest living tree species and one of the most popular herbal remedies in the world. It's a famous property of use for a wide variety of brain-related disorders — memory loss, poor concentration, mental confusion, depression, and anxiety. [63] [64]

- Bacopa monnieri has been a traditional Ayurvedic medicine for centuries for various purposes as a brain tonic to enhance memory, learning, and concentration, reduce anxiety, and treat epilepsy. It is well known as an adaptogen, a substance that moderates the negative effects of stress. It works by balancing dopamine and serotonin while reducing the stress hormone cortisol levels. [65]

- Ginger (Zingiber official) has been used for over 5,000 years as a medicinal herb in traditional Chinese and Indian Ayurvedic healing practices. Ginger is an impressive antioxidant and anti-inflammatory property. Of the 100+ compounds classified in ginger, 50 are antioxidants. Especially two unique kinds of antioxidants, shaogals, and gingerols, ensure the brain from damaging free radicals. Ginger soothes inflammation, a compromise cause for various brain-related conditions, including depression. *Ginger boosts levels of both dopamine and serotonin.*[66] [67] [68]

- Ginseng (Panax ginseng) is the typical Chinese medical herb. Its botanical name means "panacea." Ginseng can help prevent memory loss and reduce age-related mental decline. With its high antioxidant and anti-inflammatory properties, ginseng can prevent and heal many of the most severe neurological conditions, including Parkinson's, Alzheimer's, Huntington's, brain ischemia, and stroke. Ginseng is an adaptogen that increases circulation, sending better blood to all your organs. That's why we have discovered people taken for erectile dysfunction. This same structure also increases blood flow to the brain. Ginseng boosts the most significant neurotransmitters, including dopamine, serotonin, GABA, norepinephrine, and brain-derived neurotrophic factor (BDNF). [69] [70] [71] [72]

- Curcumin is consumed in Asia either as turmeric directly or as one of the culinary ingredients in food recipes. Curcumin has global recognition because of its antioxidant, anti-inflammatory, anti-cancer, and antimicrobial activities. Curcumin increases both dopamine and serotonin, two brain chemicals associated with depression. [73] Studies have found it effective for treating major neurological diseases such as Alzheimer's disease, Parkinson's disease, Multiple Sclerosis, Huntington's disease, prions disease, stroke, Down's syndrome, autism, Amyotrophic lateral sclerosis, anxiety, depression, and aging. [74]

In conclusion

Sugar addiction is like alcohol and drug addiction. It is because of a chemical imbalance in the brain.

To overcome such a severe issue, we must eat food which increases the level of dopamine and serotonin in our body with exercise, sunshine, activities that boost those brain chemicals, have a good sleep, reduce the stress in our daily life and the most important in making peace with your past, forgive people and love yourself. I hope this information helps with clarity and guideline to go in the right direction. If you are out of the track, it's ok. I have been out of track many times. You are all in, and you are out, then you learn. If you don't do all the right things at one time, it is ok, and this is normal. Come back and do it again. Again, and again. The more you practice, the more you learn. The knowledge you have more and more every day will be the wisdom that you earn, and no one can take it away from you.

I have healed from what I have learned from my reading and research. I set myself free from the past. Growing up as a Buddhist in Thailand helped me let go and be in the present moment.

I have been practicing positive affirmations, manifest, and meditation to help me heal my heart. It takes time to heal, yes! However, even though it's slow, you will get there if you do it. Slowly but surely, like a turtle!

My belief in God also helps me to get through my hard times. As I mentioned earlier, I might write another book about what's going on with me during lent in 2019.

Before subtracting anything, add something first. I asked you to add fiber, outdoor activities, and smile in chapter 2, and I asked you to write your stress relievers in chapter 3. So before stopping sugar and refined carbs, just keep adding. If you take care of your body as a whole, you will heal. In this chapter, you learn how foods and activities help to fulfill your brain chemistry: serotonin and dopamine. Did you know? Over 90% of serotonin and over 50% of dopamine are made from our gut. Let's find out more details in the next chapter.

TO-DO-LIST

- Add more vegetables and fruits to your daily intake.

- Add at least 5 activities you love.

- Get a notebook, write your negative thoughts, and transfer them to positive ones. You can learn from my book. **Daily Affirmations for Prosperity and Happiness: 500 Positive Affirmations to Reset Your Brain.**

CHAPTER 5

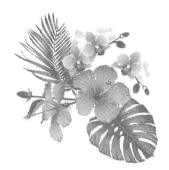

SUGAR DETOX WITH GUT MICROBIOME PRINCIPLE

You might have questions. What are you going to have for this sugar detox plan? Certainly, you will not consume sugar. So, what am I going to have? Is carbohydrate in the picture? How about fruits? Many of you might have heard some types of diet mentioned fruits make you fat. You might be confused because we have so many diet principles that claim weight loss, such as, Keto diet, Paleo diet, vegan diet, vegetarian diet, Mediterranean diet, dash diet, noom diet, Nordic diet, and the list goes on and on.

This detox program has a primary focus on your health. Once everything in your body is harmonized, the weight loss will follow as a side effect. What a side effect? I'm just kidding. You might say it's not my primary goal to pick up your book, Triya. I want to lose weight. I heard you, and I knew it very well. As a personal trainer and nutrition coach, I have worked with many people who want to lose weight and be healthy. Most people come to me for the primary goal of weight loss, but believe me, you will find harmony and balance for your body and your life during your weight loss journey. Weight loss will follow naturally once you understand how your body works and work with it, but not against it. I will show you how easy it is as I have been on this path, and it works for me, so it's your option if you follow my guidance for 21 days, or you can adopt the foundation of my detox plan and use it as your own diet. Imagine if I'm a captain who has traveled the world, and now I'm telling you how I did it successfully, including tips and tricks that I have accomplished during my journey. In this chapter, I'm going share why sugar detox with the gut microbiome principle is the key.

Fiber is the food for the gut microbiome. In chapter 2, I pointed out about 2 types of fiber. Soluble fiber and insoluble fiber. Fiber has so many health benefits, such as keeping you full longer, helping you have a regular bowel movement, stabilizing blood sugar levels, reducing fat absorption, lowering cholesterol, decreasing the risk of heart disease, supporting weight management, and feeding your gut microbiome, which is one of the master blueprints for the sugar detox plan.

In chapter 3, you learn that your brain controls your sugar addiction, and now you know how to lead the game by understanding your serotonin and dopamine, so your brain can't fool you anymore.

YOUR BRAIN IS NOT A BIG BOSS, BUT YOUR GUT IS.

Your gut controls your brain, and do you know who controls the gut? The answer is your gut microbiome. So, if you want to have everything under control, I mean everything from waking until sleeping, and 24/7. If you wish to have it all in your body, run smoothly and in harmony. You would better learn and know your little friend's "gut microbiome," and you will become the big boss of your community.

YOUR GUT MICROBIOTA HAS A MAGIC WAND.

They can do amazing work for your body, such as;

- Helping you lose weight, stop sugar craving, and overcome sugar addiction.

- Fighting COVID-19, other viruses, and pathogens by building strong immunity.

- Enhancing your mood and keeping a big smile all day long

- Preventing cancer and neurotransmitter disorders.

Gut and brain connection is not fiction, but fact.

Many studies show that your brain health and gut health affect each other in many ways. The communication system between your gut and brain is called the gut-brain axis. They communicate with each other all the time through the vagus nerve in both directions. The vagus nerve represents the major component of the nervous system, which oversees a tremendous amount of essential body functions, including control of mood, immune response, digestion, and heart rate. [75]

Your brain and your gut are again connected through neurotransmitters, the body's chemical messengers which influence mood and health. As in chapter 3, you learn about brain chemicals, dopamine and serotonin. More than 90% of serotonin and over 50% of dopamine are produced in the gut.

Do you want to wake up wonderfully and feel fantastic all day long? If so, it's better to get to know the gut microbiota and learn how to feed them the right food.

WHAT IS GUT MICROBIOTA?

If you feel lonely during the pandemic covid-19. I want to tell you; you are not alone. Every day you have someone being with you all the time, from the day you were born until the day you leave this beautiful world. You are a host of bacteria, viruses, fungi, and other microscopic living things called microorganisms or microbes. Within the human gastrointestinal (GI) tract, microbiota exists in a complex ecosystem of approximately 300 to 500 bacterial species, comprising nearly 2 million genes (the microbiome) and more than a trillion. Indeed, the number of bacteria within the gut is almost 10 times that of all the cells in the human body. That means you are more bacteria than a human. You are a host, and they live inside your body and benefit the host. When we feed them food (aka. fiber), they produce short-chain fatty acids (SCFAs) through their fermentation process. About 95% of the short-chain fatty acids in your body are: acetate (C2), butyrate (C4), propionate (C3). [78] [79]

Microbiome—the collective genomes of the micro-organisms in a particular environment

Microbiota—the community of micro-organisms themselves

WHY CAN SHORT-CHAIN FATTY ACIDS HELP YOU?

Table 1: summary

SCFA	Health benefits	Main producer
Acetate	regulates pH of the gut; controls appetite; nourishes butyrate-producing bacteria; protects against pathogens	Bifidobacteria, Lactobacillus, Akkermansia muciniphila, Prevotella spp., Ruminococcus spp.
Butyrate	energy source for colon cells; helps prevent leaky gut, anti-inflammation, anti-cancer activity, and protects the brain	Faecalibacterium prausnitzii, Eubacterium rectale, and Roseburia spp.
Propionate	regulates appetite; combats inflammation; helps protect against cancer	Bacteroidetes, Firmicutes, Lachnospiraceae
Lactate	nourishes butyrate-producing bacteria; regulates the immune system; fights opportunistic bacteria, produce vitamin B12	Lactic acid bacteria

Acetate

helps to support your gut environment and sustains other beneficial bacteria species in your colon.

Acetate is an essential regulator of the pH of your gut. It restores the gut acidic enough for your beneficial microbes to thrive and survive but prevents the bad ones from coming in and sticking around. Your gut bacteria produce a higher percentage of acetate among SCFAs. The approximate ratio of acetate, propionate, and butyrate is 60:20:20. Therefore, the production of these compounds is essential to our overall health and wellbeing.

Acetate also binds to receptors in the gut lining, where it regulates appetite and fat storage. These receptors have powerful aspects in stimulating the release of specific gut hormones, glucagon-like peptide-1 (GLP-1) and peptide YY, which regulate our appetite.

You don't feel hungry after these hormones are released by the cell in the small intestine, so you can stop snacking and taking extra calories. The acetate made from the breakdown of fiber can even help you lose weight via an increase in energy expenditure and fat oxidation.[80]

The acetate produced by bacteria, such as bifidobacteria, helps to cultivate the butyrate-producing microbes in your gut, supporting the diversity of your beneficial microorganisms. Therefore, this SCFA helps other species grow and survive, a behavior called cross-feeding.

Butyrate

is significant for our digestive system and disease prevention, including neurological conditions and cancer prevention and helping you to lose weight.

Butyrate has many functions in both our body and gut. One of its fundamental roles is a primary energy source for the cells lining the gut called "colonocytes."

Your gut lining is extremely important because it creates a barrier between your intestinal environment and the rest of your body. It stops opportunistic pathogens, toxins, and food components from getting into your blood and causing you ill. In the meantime, when the lining works effectively, it allows beneficial things like vitamins and minerals to enter the bloodstream and make their way to different parts of the body that need them. The barrier controls the opening and closing of the lining. But if these junctions cannot close, it can cause a leaky gut. But by having plenty of butyrate producers, you will have an expanded production of this SCFA, which means you'll be protected from leaky gut.

Butyrate is not only good for gut health. It's remarkable for the brain too. Butyrate works via the gut-brain axis, a two-way communication process between the two organs. Eating a high-fiber diet positively affects our nervous system, cognition, and memory. This could help prevent neurodegenerative diseases like Alzheimer's, Parkinson's, mental health disorders, and autism. [81]

Another glorious thing about the gut microbiome and fiber breakdown is its antioxidant and anticancer properties. It has an incredible way of doing it by causing rogue cells to kill themselves and prevent cancer from developing. [82] [83] It's too good to be true, right?

The study in 2018 in mice revealed a butyrate is a remarkable tool for weight loss by activating brown adipose tissue (BAT) and increasing oxidation of intracellular fatty acids. Butyrate in the gut also produces the endocrine hormones glucagon-like peptide 1 (GLP-1) and peptide YY (PYY), so it helps in reducing food intake. Thus, weight loss-enhancing strategies can be the most effective interventions for obesity-related diseases, diabetes, cardiovascular disease, insulin resistance, and nonalcoholic fatty liver disease (NAFLD). [84]

Propionate

has powerful health benefits, such as reducing fat storage, lowering cholesterol, anti-cancer, and anti-inflammatory properties.

Propionate stimulates the release of the hormone's peptide YY and GLP-1, an anti-obesity and anti-diabetic action like acetate and butyrate. Once these hormones are released, you will be satisfied with your food, and it will stop you from keeping eating and snacking. The result is that you will lose weight and lose unwanted body fat easily. These two hormones are stimulated by resistance starch (RS) through its colonic fermentation. So, it's better to eat resistant starch and not be confused about eating carbohydrates anymore.

Propionate has similar properties like butyrate that can modulate brain function and prevent a neurodegenerative disorder [85] and has anti-cancer properties. [86] The cool thing is that it makes cancer cells commit suicide, so it's preventing cancer from developing.

Lactate

is not a short-chain fatty acid, but it's produced by gut bacteria and makes valuable enhancements to your colon health.

Lactic acid bacteria or lactobacillus are the primary producers of lactate. You might have heard about food made with the benefit of *Lactobacillus,* such as yogurt, milk, cheese, and kefir products. Lactic acid bacteria have been used for centuries to ferment foods, a preparation that also preserves them.

Lactobacillus itself is a remarkable member of your gut microbiome because it helps to protect you from harm. It even releases substances to prevent pathogens in your gut. [87]

It has a significant role in your immune system. It can perform as a peacemaker for both the production of pro-and anti-inflammatory cytokines. In the gut, lactate helps to reduce inflammation. [88] So don't be surprised that taking Lactobacillus can prevent and improve symptoms of the common cold.[89] A few studies showed that L. acidophilus could help reduce the common cold symptoms in children to avoid missing school. [90] [91]

Research shows that lactate can increase brain function. They also support fewer symptoms of depression and treat panic disorder (PD). Increasing your fiber consumption can have many effective benefits for your mood and brain health. [92] [93]

AMAZING GUT-MADE VITAMIN B12 AND MORE

Lactic acid bacteria are vital organisms in producing vitamin B12, which cannot be synthesized by either animals, plants, or fungi. Bifidobacterial are primary producers of folate, a vitamin involved in vital host metabolic processes, including DNA synthesis and repair.

Additional vitamins, which gut microbiota have been shown to synthesize in humans, include vitamin K both K1 (phylloquinone) and K2 (menaquinone), the B-group (or B-complex) vitamins include thiamine (B1), riboflavin (B2), niacin (B3), pyridoxine (B6), pantothenic acid (B5), biotin (B7 or H), folate (B11–B9 or M) and cobalamin (B12). [94] [95] B-group vitamins, normally present in many foods, are easily removed or destroyed during cooking and food processing, so insufficient intake is common in many societies. [96]

Now you know our gut microbiota has tremendous benefits to your health. You have had them since you were born, but several environmental factors have shaped the microbiota, including geographic location, surgery, smoking, depression, living arrangements (urban or rural), and antibiotics. Antibiotic treatment disrupts both short- and long-term microbial balance, including decreases in the richness and diversity of the community. [97]

HOW TO INCREASE GUT MICROBIOME DIVERSITY

Master key to success

PREBIOTICS + PROBIOTICS = POSTBIOTICS

What are prebiotics?

Prebiotics are supplements or foods containing non-digestible ingredients that stimulate indigenous bacteria's growth and activity.

What are probiotics?

Probiotics are supplements or foods that contain viable microorganisms that alter the host's microflora.

What are postbiotics?

Postbiotics are non-viable bacterial products or metabolic byproducts from probiotic microorganisms with biological activity in the host. [98]

Prebiotic, a fancy name for vegetables, whole grains, fruit, and nuts. You do not need to spend money to buy supplements if you eat enough of them, and in this plan, you will have enough of them. However, adding supplements is optional, and I will tell you later if you need it.

Probiotics are a combination of live beneficial bacteria and yeasts that live in your body. You can find foods that have been fermented, such as yogurt, kimchi, and sauerkraut.

To have the most post biotics, which is beneficial to your body. You will consume food that feeds the microbes, so then they will survive and thrive. Once they get the food, they will be happy and multiply more and more for the community. Different microbes prefer different types of food. It's a good idea to have a variety of whole grains, fruits, and vegetables. The nasty microbe will ask for more sugary or fatty food. In contrast, a good microbe will order a good choice of food. Good microbes do so many wonderful things to your body. Once you feed them, then they will give you the benefits. Therefore, it's better to feed the good ones, so they don't die off, but let the bad ones die off. It's a good idea, right?

The prebiotic and probiotic foods that heal your gut and support your microbiome will help you lose weight automatically. Yes, you heard it right; you don't need to do anything extra and no need for an extended period of exercise or huff and puff, but you still lose weight or maintain the one you prefer when your gut is in optimum condition, and your microbiome is balanced.

First, I would like to introduce you to "the dietary fiber" in depth. Now I don't talk about fiber that helps you go to the bathroom in the morning, but I'm going to introduce you to the most beneficial fiber that helps you lose weight, have more energy throughout the day, boost the immune system, get rid of the new generation problems such as obesity, heart disease, diabetes, autoimmune disease, cancer, and allergy.

A classification of dietary fiber is often based on its water solubility, viscosity, and fermentability. The intestinal microbiota ferment of soluble fiber to SCFA, mainly acetate, propionate, and butyrate.

However, insoluble fiber is essential because it helps you go to the bathroom and keep the gut in a healthy and balanced environment.

Fiber has 2 main types:

First is oligosaccharides, and the second is Polysaccharides.[99] Do not worry about this fancy name. I just added it here for you to see the complete picture.

1. Oligosaccharide is soluble but less viscous and fermentable and includes resistant oligosaccharides (RO). It has 4 types:

- Fructooligosaccharides or FOS
- Galactooligosaccharides or GOS
- Resistant dextrins
- Polydextrose

2. Polysaccharides are further classified into non-starch polysaccharides (NSP) and resistant starch (RS)

2.1 non-starch polysaccharides (NSP) vary to a large extent, with some being soluble, viscous, and fermentable, while others are not. It has 6 types:

- Cellulose
- Hemicelluloses (heteroxylans)
- Mannans and heteromannans
- Pectin
- Inulin and fructans
- Other hydrocolloids

2.2 Resistance Starch (RS) is not soluble and viscous and only partly fermentable. It has 5 types:

- RS type 1
- RS type 2
- RS type 3
- RS type 4
- RS type 5

I mentioned this fancy name because you can come back to look at it as a reference when I share the secret of a powerful prebiotic.

> *Sweet surprise*
>
> *Research showed that two short-chain fructans - oligofructose and inulin are a simulator of the Human Intestinal Microbial Ecosystem (SHIME) in vitro model. Inulin with longer chain lengths such as chicory has a slower breakdown, more beneficial changes in the microbial community (both proximal and distal), higher acetate production, and higher bifidogenic effect in the distal colon than oligofructose.* [100]

How to increase your gut microbiome diversity

I.   Natural prebiotic food

The most common prebiotics are oligosaccharides found in human milk. The benefit of breastfeeding is suitable for both mother and the baby and the baby's gut microbiome because breast milk has a natural prebiotic.

Once the baby gets bigger, they can chew and eat food by themselves. Nature provides you with natural prebiotics that comes with whole food plant-based.

Not all fiber is prebiotic. Fiber can help you go to the bathroom and help you have good digestion, but food classified as prebiotic can help you lose weight, boost your immune system, and fight COVID-19 or any other new virus that you may have faced in the future. Prebiotics is the foods that feed your good gut microbiome, and they also produce more good gut bacteria; Bifidobacteria and Lactobacilli.

(Bifidobacteria live in the GI tract of healthy human adults and have a strong affinity to ferment select oligosaccharides, making them a standard marker for prebiotic capacity.

Lactobacilli have been shown to downregulate mucosal inflammation in the GI tract. Lactobacilli play a role in helping digest lactose for lactose-intolerant individuals, alleviate constipation, improve irritable bowel syndrome (IBS) symptoms, and help prevent traveler's diarrhea.

Prebiotics reduce a bad bacteria population, decrease allergy risk, increase calcium absorption, decrease protein fermentation, affect gut barrier permeability and production of beneficial metabolites. [101]

SUPERFOOD FOR YOUR GUT MICROBIOME

1. Apples

You have heard, "An apple a day keeps the doctor away." An apple is full of vitamins, minerals, fiber, and antioxidants. The various antioxidants in apples, such as flavonoids, quercetin, catechin, and chlorogenic acid found in apples, are compounds that have been shown to reduce inflammation, protect heart health, antiviral, anticancer, and antidepressant effects.[102] [103] Apples contain 2%–3% fiber. They are rich in insoluble fiber, including cellulose and hemicellulose, with pectin as the primary soluble fiber. Apple pectin and polyphenols in apples could promote healthy gut microbiota increase butyrate, a short-chain fatty acid that feeds beneficial gut bacteria and decreases the number of harmful bacteria. [104] Pectin fiber from apples also has cholesterol-lowering properties and beneficial effects on glucose metabolism, suppressing weight gain and fat accumulation. [105] [106]

2. Asparagus

is a popular vegetable that contains inulin. Inulin is a type of plant fiber found in many plant-based foods. It's a soluble fiber that feeds the friendly bacteria in the gut, such as Bifidobacteria and Lactobacillus[107], and it helps curb hunger and increases the feeling of fullness after meals. The human body doesn't make digestive enzymes that can break down inulin. So, it can't be digested in the stomach or small intestine, but it moves through the digestive system to the large intestine, where it feeds the gut bacteria. However, if you have IBS (Irritable bowel syndrome), avoid this type of fiber.

3. Bananas (unripe)

have a small amount of inulin, rich in vitamins and minerals. Green bananas are high in resistant starch (RS Type 2). RS is fermented in the large intestine by butyrate-producing bacteria, including *Eubacterium rectale and Bifidobacterium species.* The SCFA butyrate is essential for maintaining the health and integrity of the gastrointestinal tract and may play a role in modulating glucose and lipid homeostasis, resulting in the control of body weight and insulin sensitivity. [108]

4. Burdock roots

Burdock (Arctium lappa) is native to northeast Asia and some countries in Europe. It belongs to the Asteraceae family and chicory roots,

Jerusalem artichoke, and yacon tubers. The roots of this family are recognized by their low starch levels and high amounts of oligosaccharides and fructan fiber, which are prebiotic which support the growth of healthy bacteria in the digestive tract such as lactobacilli and bifidobacteria strains.[109]

5. Cacao or Cocoa

The cocoa bean also called the cacao bean, is Theobroma cacao's dried and fermented seed. Cocoa beans are the basis of chocolate, and it's so delicious.

Cocoa powder is made by crushing cocoa beans and removing the fat, and cocoa butter is the fat part. The powder is convenient to add to smoothies, yogurt, dessert, pancakes, or just simply a delicious cup of hot chocolate.

Cocoa and its products are rich sources of polyphenols, such as flavanols. These compounds exert antioxidant and anti-inflammatory activities. Cocoa polyphenols are prebiotic, and they enhance the growth of beneficial gut bacteria, such as Lactobacillus and Bifidobacterium, while reducing the number of bad ones such as Clostridium pathogenic species. [110]

6. Chicory root

is famous for its coffee-like flavor and high antioxidant, anticancer, anti-inflammatory, antiparasitic properties, and protection against liver damage. 68% of chicory root fiber comes from the prebiotic fiber inulin. Inulin in chicory root helps relieve constipation and improve digestion and bowel function. A study on blood glucose, lipid metabolism, and fecal properties found that it helps prevent diabetes by raising adiponectin levels (a protein that helps control blood glucose levels). [111]

7. Dandelion greens and Dandelion root

The root of dandelion contains inulin, which includes fructooligosaccharides (FOS). FOS is a complex carbohydrate; its intake benefits bifidobacteria, eliminating pathogens in the gastrointestinal tract and increasing friendly bacteria in your gut, reducing constipation, and boosting your immune system. This is one magical plant on earth that can help you lose weight. It also has anti-diabetic, anti-inflammatory, antioxidant, and anticancer effects. [112] [113]

8. Flaxseeds

or linseeds contain the essential omega-3 fatty acid alpha-linolenic acid (ALA) and lignans, a type of phytoestrogen, a group of compounds linked to a reduced risk of heart disease, developing osteoporosis, and breast cancer. Lignans also have antioxidant properties that protect cells from damage. It has an excellent source of high-quality plant protein, and it is an excellent source of soluble fiber.

Flaxseed's fiber is a prebiotic and fermented by gut microbiota to short-chain fatty acids. It promotes healthy gut bacteria, reduces the amount of dietary fat you digest and absorb, and helps with regular bowel movements. [114] [115]

9. Garlic

Garlic has so many health benefits, including preventing gastrointestinal diseases, antioxidant, anti-inflammatory, and lower cholesterol properties. One of the major components, garlic fructan (GF), was evaluated for its prebiotic effectiveness on human intestinal microflora, and it promotes the growth of beneficial Bifidobacteria in the gut. It also prevents harmful bacteria from growing. [116] [117]

10. Konjac root

is a tuber, a vegetable grown underground, like the potato. The plant has been used for centuries in Asia as food and medicine. Flour made from this plant contains 70-90% glucomannan fiber, which has health benefits for anti-obesity, regulation in lipid metabolism, laxative effect, anti-diabetic, and anti-inflammatory. [118] Konjac glucomannan is prebiotic that increases the levels of short-chain fatty acids (SCFAs) in the colon.[119] [120] You can find them in the food, such as shirataki noodles and miracle noodles. You can add the shirataki noodles in curry, stir-fry, and any food you wish. It is tasteless and absorbs the flavor and all sauces very well. I love to add them to Thai green curry or even Tom yum.

11. Jerusalem artichoke

The Jerusalem artichoke — also known as the sunchoke, sun root, or earth apple — is part of the sunflower family. It's one of God's gifts because this medical plant not only helps increase the friendly bacteria in your colon with inulin and promotes more excellent digestive health but also aids in the absorption of minerals in your large intestine.

This sunflower-like plant has anti-diabetic, anti-cancer, anti-fungal, and anti-constipation properties. It can help with body mass-reducing, boost metabolism, help strengthen your immune system, help lower cholesterol, triglycerides, and glucose levels. It's great for weight loss, detoxification (e.g., alcohol, heavy metals, and radiation), and even prevents certain metabolic disorders. [121]

12. Jicama

is low in calories and high in Vitamin C, enhancing the immune system and insulin sensitivity and lowering blood sugar levels. It contains the prebiotic fiber inulin, which significantly benefits gut diversity and helps improve digestive health.[122] [123]

13. Leeks

come from the allium family of garlic and onion. They have a sweet, oniony flavor that adds depth to soups, stews, curry, stir-fried, and any delicious dish. They are nutrient-dense vegetables high in vitamin K and high in inulin that promote healthy gut bacteria and help break down fat.

14. Onions

are rich in fructans and fructooligosaccharides (FOS), which help boost your immune system by increasing nitric oxide production in cells and good gut bacteria such as Bifidobacteria and Lactobacilli.[124] [125]

Onion is the vegetable that you should eat every day. Onions are rich in the flavonoid and quercetin, which gives onions antioxidant, anticancer, anti-allergic effect, antibiotic and anti-inflammatory properties.[126] [127] [128]

15. Seaweed

or sea vegetables are forms of algae that grow in the sea. Seaweeds are an excellent source of nutrients, such as proteins, vitamins, minerals, and dietary fiber. They have amazing health benefits such as antioxidant, anti-inflammatory, anti-cancer, anti-obesity, and anti-diabetic properties thanks to polyphenols, polysaccharides, and sterols compounds. They also have a higher proportion of essential fatty acids as eicosapentaenoic (EPA) and docosahexaenoic (DHA) fatty acids, we know as Omega-3. [129]

Seaweeds are soluble and insoluble fiber, and 50–85% are water-soluble fiber. Studies showed the polysaccharides found in seaweed could increase the production of short-chain fatty acids (SCFA), which helps to improve gut health. [130]

16. Wheat bran

is rich in AXOS prebiotic (Arabinoxylan Oligosaccharide). A unique fiber from wheat bran has been shown to boost healthy Bifidobacteria in the gut. [131] [132] [133] Bifidobacteria are a large group of bacteria that live in the intestines. Bifidobacteria are used as probiotics and medicine. It is used for constipation, diarrhea, an intestinal disorder called irritable bowel syndrome (IBS), to prevent the common cold or flu, and many other conditions. So don't be afraid to eat whole wheat bread or products that are made from whole wheat flour anymore because many studies showed wheat bran contains high levels of the *hemicellulose arabinoxylan*, which can be used by the bacteria inhabiting the microbiota and found that the effect of wheat/rye bread intake was most pronounced on butyrate. Therefore, they are also suitable for digestion, gut health, and brain health. [134] [135] [136]

17. Yacon root

is a tuber vegetable, just like potatoes. It contains fructooligosaccharides (FOS), inulin, and phenolic compounds, which promote the growth of good gut bacteria such as lactobacillus and bifidobacteria in the colon, enhancing mineral absorption, boosting the immune system and gastrointestinal metabolism. It also plays an essential role in regulating serum cholesterol and lipid metabolism. As a result, glycemic levels, body weight, and colon cancer risk can be reduced. [137] [138]

18. Resistant starches (RS)

Is a portion of starch that cannot be digested by amylases in the small intestine and passes to the colon to be fermented by microbiota.

There are 5 types of resistant starch.

RS 1 Starch is synthesized in the endosperm of cereal grains or seeds, and starch granules are surrounded by protein matrix and cell wall material. These physical structures hinder the digestibility of starch and reduce the glycemic response. We can find RS1 in grains, seeds, and legumes. Examples of type 1 resistant starch include bread made with whole or coarse ground kernels of grains and pasta made with durum wheat extrusion.

RS 2 Uncooked potato starch, green banana starch, ginkgo starch, and high-amylose maize starch, which display the B- or C-type polymorph, are resistant to enzymatic hydrolysis.

RS 3 is retrograded amylose and starch. For example, potatoes and rice are cooked and then cooled in the refrigerator or near refrigeration temperatures (4–5°C or 32 - 41 Fahrenheit). The cooling turns some of the digestible starches into resistant starches via retrogradation.

RS 4 is modified starch, formed either by cross-linking or chemical derivatives. For example, cross-linked starch and octenyl succinate starch.

RS 5 When starch interacts with lipids, amylose, and long branch chains of amylopectin from single-helical complexes with fatty acids and fatty alcohols. For example, stearic acid-complexed high-amylose starch. [139]

When resistant starch passes through the small intestine undigested then reaches to colon, the bacteria digest resistant starches.

They form several compounds, including gases and short-chain fatty acids, mostly butyrate. [140]

> *Sweet surprise*
>
> *Do you know polyphenols have prebiotic properties? Read more in chapter 7.*

19. High β-glucan food group

Foods with high β-glucan levels such as barley, oat, sorghum, triticale, wheat, and rice. Also found in foods like mushrooms, algae, and other marine plants. Beta-glucan is a prebiotic fiber that promotes the growth of friendly bacteria in your digestive tracts, such as Lactobacillus and Pediococcus species. It also could enhance the growth rate and the lactic acid production of microbes. B-glucans have been proven to strengthen the immune system and beneficial effects on obesity, cardiovascular diseases, diabetes, and cholesterol levels.[141] [142] [143] [144]

In conclusion, you can see if you know what to eat and feed your gut bacteria. You can get many benefits from them without worrying about weight gain or health problems. I am sure you will enjoy the delicious recipes on the 21 days sugar detox with add-on prebiotic for your health and keep your weight off quickly.

Next,

II. Natural probiotics food

The term probiotic is derived from the Latin preposition "pro," which means "for," and the Greek word "biotic," meaning "life." Probiotic means "for life." The Food and Agriculture Organization of the United Nations (FAO) and the World Health Organization (WHO) define probiotics as "live microorganisms that, when administered in adequate amounts, confer a health benefit on the host"

Probiotics are beneficial microbes that bring many powerful benefits throughout your body from head to toes and take care of your health and beauty from inside out.

You can simply take probiotics from supplements, but you can also have them from delicious, fermented foods.

16 PROBIOTIC FOODS THAT BOOST YOUR GUT HEALTH

1. Acidophilus Milk

Acidophilus milk has been referred to either as milk fermented with L. acidophilus or as unfermented milk containing L. acidophilus. [145] Acidophilus milk or probiotic dairy food products represent the largest segment of the functional food market in Europe, Japan, and Australia. The fermented milk in the market today represents ~€ 63.2 billion, with North America, Europe, and Asia accounting for 77% of the market. The development and consumption of functional foods, or foods that promote health beyond providing essential nutrition, are on the rise. Currently, more than 100 probiotic fermented milk products may be found in the market, of which Yakult, Actimel, and LC-1 are the most known. [146] Studies have shown that consumption of milk products containing L. acidophilus has the potential for

1) Preventing or controlling intestinal infections.

2) Improving lactose digestion in persons classified as lactose maldigestion.

3) Helping control serum cholesterol levels

4) Exerting anti-cancer activity. [147]

2. Kefir

Kefir and acidophilus milk have live cultures but vary in which bacteria and how many they have. Acidophilus milk contains Lactobacillus acidophilus. It may also include Bifidobacterium bifidum. Kefir contains much more.

Kefir is a complex fermented dairy product created through the symbiotic fermentation of milk by lactic acid bacteria and yeasts contained within an exopolysaccharide and protein complex called a **kefir grain**. Kefir is traditionally made with cow's milk, but it can be made from other sources such as goat, sheep, buffalo, or soy milk. Kefir grains, resembling miniature cauliflower florets and comprising a wide variety of symbiotic yeasts, *Lactobacillus, Lactococcus, Streptococcus, and Leuconostoc*, are added to milk in kefir manufacturing. After that, they can multiply from 24 to 56 stains in the kefir grain and 22 to 61 strains in kefir milk, making them a rich and diverse probiotic source. For this reason, kefir is a more powerful probiotic than yogurt and acidophilus milk.

The word "kefir" is derived from the Turkish word "keyif", which means "feeling good" after its ingestion.

Kefir has been associated with a range of health benefits such as cholesterol metabolism and angiotensin-converting enzyme (ACE) inhibition, antimicrobial activity, tumor suppression, increased speed of wound healing, modulation of the immune system, including the alleviation of allergy and asthma, effecting as yogurt in reducing expired hydrogen and flatulence lactose intolerant adults as well as has a big impact on the Gastrointestinal Tract (GIT). [148] [149]

3. Kimchi

Kimchi is a traditional Korean food manufactured by fermenting vegetables with probiotic lactic acid bacteria (LAB) or Lactobacillus kimchi. Many bacteria are involved in kimchi fermentation, but LAB becomes dominant while the putrefactive bacteria are suppressed during the salting of baechu cabbage and the fermentation. The major ingredients of kimchi are napa cabbage or known as Chinese cabbage, and other healthy functional foods such as garlic, ginger, black pepper, cinnamon, onion, mustard, and red pepper powder. Kimchi can be made from different vegetables such as daikon, scallion, cucumber, ponytail radish leek, watercress, and carrot.

Napa cabbage has a high nutrients value, and it contains vitamins A and C, 34 amino acids with threonine, arginine, γ-aminobutyric acid, alanine, asparagine, serine, and glutamic acid being quantitatively the most important, 10 mineral elements among which Calcium, Magnesium, Vitamin K in higher relative abundance, lutein and β-carotene as the major carotenoids. The raw materials used in preparing kimchi result in increased nutritional value, for example, the high levels of vitamins such as vitamin C, b-carotene, vitamin B complex, minerals such as sodium, calcium, potassium, iron, and vitamin P (known as flavonoids). It is also an excellent source of dietary fiber and other functional components such as allyl compounds, gingerol, capsaicin, isothiocyanate, and chlorophyll.

Kimchi is rich in several phytochemicals such as indole compounds, b-sitosterol, benzyl isothiocyanate, and thiocyanate, which showed that kimchi has anti-cancer anti-obesity, anti-constipation, anti-aging, antioxidative and probiotic properties. It promotes gut health, brain health, and skin health, boosts immunity, reduces bad cholesterol, and prevents blood clots. [150]

> *People all around the world know kimchi, but few people know that apart from kimchi, it is a functional food. Korea has more fermented foods, such as;*
>
> *- Chongkukjang, a fermented product manufactured by short-term fermentation of boiled soybean seeds using Bacillus subtilis in rice straw.*
>
> *- Doenjang is traditionally used in Korea as a basic seasoning. It is produced by the fermentation of cooked and crushed soybean seeds or blocks, Meju, by naturally occurring bacteria and fungi with brine in a container such as a porcelain pot. It has been consumed for centuries as a protein and flavoring ingredient in Korea.*
>
> *- Ganjang is a kind of Korean soybean sauce made from fermented soybeans. It contains 15–20% salt, 50–70% water, free sugars, isoflavone, peptides, and organic acids produced from the soybeans during the fermentation process.*
>
> *- Gochujang is a fermented paste made of red chili powder, glutinous rice powder, pureed soybeans and salt, seasonings like garlic and onion, sweetened with a bit of sugar syrup, and fermented for a long period in designed earthen vessels. It is an essential part of Korean cuisine. It is used in almost all Korean foods like bibimbap, noodles, etc.* [151]

4. Kombucha

Kombucha tea is a slightly sweet, slightly acidic refreshing beverage consumed worldwide. It is obtained from an infusion of tea leaves by the fermentation of a symbiotic association of bacteria and yeasts forming "tea fungus." It can be prepared with black tea or green tea. However, the research found that kombucha prepared with green tea has a higher concentration of lactic acid than kombucha prepared from black tea.

Kombucha was first used in East Asia for its healing benefits. It originated in northeast China (Manchuria), where it was prized during the Tsin Dynasty ("Ling Chi"), about 220 B.C., for its detoxifying and energizing properties. In 414 A.D., the physician Kombu brought the tea fungus to Japan, and he used it to cure the digestive problems of Emperor Inkyo. As trade routes expanded, kombucha (former trade name "Mo-Gu") found its way first into Russian (as Chaini Grib, Cainii kvass, Japonskigrib, Kambucha, Jsa Kvaska) and then into other eastern European areas, appearing in Germany (as Heldenpilz, Kombucha Schwamm) around the turn of the 20th century. During World War II, this beverage was again introduced into Germany. In the 1950s, it arrived in France and France-dominated North Africa, where its consumption became quite popular. The habit of drinking fermented tea became acceptable throughout Europe until World War II, which brought widespread shortages of tea leaves and sugar. In the postwar years, Italian society's passion for the beverage (called "Funko Chinese") peaked in the 1950s. In the 1960s, science researchers in Switzerland reported drinking kombucha was beneficial as eating yogurt and kombucha's popularity increased. Today, kombucha is sold worldwide in retail food stores in different flavors, and kombucha culture is sold on several online shopping websites.

Tea fungus or kombucha is the common name given to a symbiotic growth of acetic acid bacteria and osmophilic yeast species in a zoogleal mat, which must be cultured in sugared tea. Tea fungus is not a mushroom, as you might have heard. The exact microbial composition of kombucha cannot be given because it varies with many species. An investigation by Marsh in 2014 showed that the dominant bacteria in 5 kombucha samples (2 from Canada and one each from Ireland, the United States, and the United Kingdom) belong to *Gluconacetobacter* (over 85% in most samples) and *Lactobacillus* (up to 30%) species. *Acetobacter* was determined in a tiny number (lower than 2%).

Studies show kombucha has many health benefits, such as antimicrobial, antioxidant, anticancer, anti-inflammatory, and liver detoxification. [152] [153]

5. Koumiss

Koumiss (also spelled Kumis, kumiss, or kumys) is a fermented dairy product traditionally made from mare's milk or donkey milk. Koumiss is a dairy product similar to kefir but is produced from a liquid starter culture, in contrast to the solid kefir "grains." Because mare's milk contains more sugars than cow's or goat's milk, kumis has a higher alcohol content than kefir. Koumiss is in its category of alcoholic drinks because it is made neither from fruit nor grain. Technically, it is closer to wine than to beer because the fermentation occurs directly from sugars, as in wine. Kumis is usually served cold or chilled. It contains 2% alcohol, 0.5-1.5% lactic acid, 2-4% milk sugar, and 2% fat, and it tastes like sour ayran.

This beverage is an ancient beverage. In his 5th-century BC history, Herodotus describes the Scythians' processing of mare's milk. Archaeological investigations of the Botai culture (c. 3700–3100 BC) of ancient Kazakhstan have revealed traces of milk in bowls from the site of Botai. [154] Koumiss is also widely produced in Russia, Kazakhstan, in Western Asia. In Mongolia, it has been adopted as the national drink known as Airag.

Studies in April 2020 have revealed the diversity of lactic acid bacteria in koumiss. 119 bacterial and 36 yeast species were identified among the 14 koumiss samples. The dominant bacterial species in koumiss were Lactobacillus helveticus, Lactobacillus kefiranofaciens, Lactococcus lactis, Lactococcus raffinolactis, and Citrobacter freundii. [155]

Koumiss has similar health benefits as kefir. They are rich probiotic foods for human consumption. Besides their probiotic nature, they possess a wide range of health benefits such as antibacterial and antifungal, antioxidant properties, regulating immunity, maintaining a healthy gastrointestinal system, controlling cholesterol, and sugar levels, regulating blood pressure, helping to get rid of lactose intolerance, inducing the production of some essential vitamins such as vitamins A, B1, B2, B12, D, E, C and it also has a protective effect against brain and kidney alterations produced by mercury toxicity. [156] [157] [158] It's difficult to find in the USA, but don't be disappointed because this drink can help you increase robustness, energy, and weight gain.

6. Mil-Mil

Mil-Mil is a Japan-originated fermented dairy product. A mixture of Bifidobacterium bifidum, Bifidobacterium breve, and Lb. Acidophilus cultures are used in the production. The Yakult Honsha company in Japan developed it. The product is enriched with small glucose, fructose, and carrot juice. Hence, it is rich in provitamin A. Mil-Mil can also be eaten as soup.

7. Miru-Miru

Miru-Miru is a dairy product made with a mix of L. casei, L. acidophilus, and Bifidobacterium breve and is produced in Japan. [159]

8. Miso

is a traditional Japanese condiment comprising a thick paste made from soybeans that have been fermented with salt and a koji starter. The starter has the *Aspergillus oryzae fungus*.

This paste is most regularly used in miso soup, and it can make sauces, spreads, soup stock, pickled vegetables, and meat. Miso comes from many varieties, such as white, brown, yellow, and red. Miso is a terrific source of protein and fiber. It is also rich in vitamins, minerals, and plant compounds, including vitamin K, manganese, and copper.

Miso has been identified to have health benefits such as reducing cardiovascular disease risk, decreasing the total and LDL cholesterol, [160] and inhibiting breast cancer.[161]

9. Natto

is another traditional Japanese dish comprising fermented soybean products, like miso. It has a bacterial strain called *Bacillus subtilis* and is described by a slimy, stringy, and sticky texture. Natto is rich in protein and vitamin K2, powerful for bone and cardiovascular health. Studies showed natto has a tremendous beneficial effect on bone health in elderly men, [162], as well as help prevent postmenopausal bone loss. [163] [164] In animal studies in 2020 also found Bacillus subtilis–based probiotics increase bone growth by inhibiting inflammation.[165]

10. Pickles

Pickles are cucumbers that have been preserved in brine or vinegar. For health purposes and live probiotics, choose simply fermented kind, where vinegar wasn't used in the pickling process. Sea salt and water solution feed the growth of good bacteria, and it may make sour pickles help improve your digestion.

They are an excellent source of vitamin K, an essential nutrient for blood clotting, and low in calories. However, keep in mind that they are also high in sodium.

I also make my own recipes for watermelon rind. The most outstanding health benefits are its ability to enhance the appearance of the skin, lower blood pressure, promote weight loss, strengthen the immune system, minimize symptoms of morning sickness in pregnant women, and increase sexual performance and libido in men.

11. Sauerkraut

is one of the most common and oldest forms of preserving cabbage since the 4th century BC. It contains a large quantity of lactic acid and tyramines and is rich in fiber, vitamins C, K, and B, iron, and manganese. It has few calories but note that it's also high in sodium. [166] Choose raw unpasteurized sauerkraut so you will get the benefit of probiotics but not from the pasteurized one because the live and active bacteria would kill by this process. You can also find raw types of sauerkraut online too.

Sauerkraut is popular in many countries, especially in Europe. However, several fermented fruits and vegetable products (Sauerkraut, Kimchi, Gundruk, Khalpi, Sinki, etc.) have a long history of human nutrition from ancient ages. They are associated with the several social aspects of different communities. Lactic acid fermentation increases the shelf life of fruits and vegetables, enhances several beneficial properties, including nutritional value and flavors, and reduces toxicity. Fermented fruits and vegetables can be used as a potential source of probiotics as they harbor several lactic acid bacteria, such as *Lactobacillus plantarum, L. pentosus, L. brevis, L. acidophilus, L. fermentum, Leuconostoc fallax, and L. mesenteroides.* [167]

Examples of traditional fermented fruits and vegetables, which are used in various parts of the world.

- China has Paocai, Yan-taozih

- India has Gundruk, Inziangsang, Sinki, Soidon

- Indonesia has Sayur asin

- Italy has Olive

- Japan has Nozawana-Zuke, Sunki

- Korea has Kimchi

- Malaysia has Tempoyak

- Nepal has Khalpi, and Sinki

- Philippines has Burong mustasa

- Spain has Olive

- Taiwan has Jiang-gua, Pobuzihi, Suan-tsai, Yan-dong-gua, Yan-jiang, Yan-taozih, Yan-tsai-shin

- Thailand has Pak-Gard-Dong, Pak-sian-dong

- Vietnam has Ca muoi, Dhamuoi, Dua muoi

So, if you don't like sauerkraut, you still can enjoy other types of fruits and vegetables fermented according to the cuisine or your taste buds.

12. Some kinds of cheese

If you are a cheese lover, you recognize they are different in taste and texture. Not all cheeses are created equal. Even though most types of cheese are fermented, it doesn't mean that all of them have probiotics.

Good bacteria survive the aging process in some cheese, such as;

- **Cheddar cheese,** a viable delivery food for probiotics; Lactobacillus casei will survive during the process and storage. It also helps protect cells against the very low pH that will be encountered during stomach transit. [168] Another study found that cheddar cheese is an excellent vehicle for various commercial probiotics since Bifidobacterium spp, Lactobacillus casei, Lactobacillus paracasei, and Lactobacillus rhamnosus survive. [169] A new study in 2020 mentioned that Lactococcus spp. Dominated Cheddar cheese (27 to 76%). [170]

- **Cottage cheese** is another type of milk product that research found the bacteria Lactobacillus plantarum Lb41 able to survive during the process. [171] [172]

- **Gouda** as the studies in 2014 they added probiotic Lactobacillus acidophilus, Lactobacillus casei, Lactobacillus paracasei, and bifidobacterium animalis subsp. lactis to full-fat, reduced-fat, and low-fat Cheddar cheeses. Probiotic bacteria can survive throughout the cheese-making and aging process. [173]

- **Kurt cheese or Kazakhstan cheese** is a traditional product that belongs to the Kazakh culture. It is made by drying fermented milk, from which yogurt is also obtained. Kurt is a versatile treasure of nomadic people's wisdom. There are varieties of names for this cheese, for example, aaruul in Mongolia, kashk in Iran, chortan in Armenia. The milk for making Kurt is obtained from sheep or mares, and the entire Kurt-making process requires the entire family group, with each person playing a unique role. This protein-packed and calcium-rich snack accompanied travelers along the Silk Road and beyond.

A study in 2017 found across the Kazakhstan cheese samples, 238 bacterial species belonging to 14 phyla and 140 genera were identified. Lactococcus lactis (28.93%), Lactobacillus helveticus (26.43%), Streptococcus thermophilus (12.18%), and Lactobacillus delbrueckii (12.15%) were the dominant bacterial species for these samples. [174] That is amazing, isn't it?

- **Maasdam** is a traditional, semi-hard Dutch cheese made from cow's milk. It is aged for at least 4 weeks; The cheese was created in the early 1990s as an alternative to more expensive Swiss Emmental cheese.

- **Mozzarella,** probiotic Lactobacillus paracasei ssp. Paracasei LBC-1 (LBC-1e) was added to part-skim mozzarella cheese and could survive during the heat treatment that is called the pasta filata process. [175]

- **Parmesan** is one of the aged cheeses that found over 10 species of bacteria. They have the dominance of Lactobacillus and Streptococcus in the average parmesan cheese. Pilot studies also found that Bifidobacterium mongoliense strains can colonize the human gut with parmesan cheese, a process that can be enhanced by cow milk consumption.

- **Parmigiano Reggiano** is a hard Italian cheese produced from cow's milk and aged at least 12 months. It is characterized by positive nutritional qualities. It is considered a "functional food" according to the definition given by the European Unit. [176]

A probiotic prospective study found 3 Lactobacillus rhamnosus strains at the end of the ripening of Parmigiano Reggiano cheese. [177] Another study related to the microbial composition of NWCs (Natural whey cultures) used for manufacturing Parmigiano Reggiano and Grana Padano was found that Lactobacillus helveticus, Streptococcus thermophilus, and Lactobacillus delbrueckii subsp. lactis form the core microbiome of these cultures. [178] The probiotic nature of Parmigiano Reggiano and its use in the prevention of intestinal and extraintestinal diseases at all ages, from infants to the elderly. Another important characteristic of Italian hard-cooked cheese is the total absence of lactose. Based on the standards of the European Commission (April 2003), Parmigiano Reggiano can be defined as 'lactose-free' products because they contain lactose in amounts no higher than 0.10 mg per 100 kcal of product. The Parmigiano Reggiano cheese has certain oligosaccharides, i.e., short-chain non-digestible carbohydrates with a possible prebiotic effect. They stimulate the multiplication of existing beneficial strains (bifidobacteria and lactobacilli) and induce local and systemic effects helpful for the host.[179] The oligosaccharides are also involved in many cellular recognition processes and have many biological activities, including immunostimulatory, anti-inflammatory, antiviral, and immunological functions. [180]

- **Pecorino di Carmasciano or Carmasciano** is an Italian cheese of the Pecorino family of cheeses made from sheep's milk. The study found the dominant species after cheese digestion could be related to the Lactobacillus plantarum and Lactobacillus casei groups. [181]

- **Provolone** is an Italian cheese made from cow's milk that originates in Southern Italy, and it is a cousin of mozzarella. Both are made in pasta filata, which means "spun paste" in Italian. 72-85% of Streptococcus was observed to be the most abundant organism in provolone, and in swiss cheese, 60 to 67% Streptococcus was observed.[182]

- **Swiss Gruyère cheese** is made from raw cow's milk, and it is known as one of the finest cheeses for baking and melting cheese, like in fondu. This hard, yellow Swiss cheese originated in the cantons of Fribourg, Vaud, Neuchâtel, Jura, and Berne in Switzerland. It is named after the town of Gruyères. A study found the diversity and abundance of Lactobacillus helveticus strain from the Swiss Gruyère cheese. Further study also found Streptococcus thermophilus and Lactobacillus delbrueckii subsp. Lactis. [183] So, you know that diversity is good for your gut by now.

13. Tempeh (or tempe) is a traditional Indonesian fermented food. Yellow seed soybeans are most popular to use as raw material, but you can also use black beans and kidney beans. Now, tempeh is popular all around the world among vegetarians and vegans. It has vitamin B12 and is a significant source of complete protein. That means it has all nine of the essential amino acids your body needs for healthy bones and muscles. During the soaking process of soybeans for tempeh fermentation, not only B12 was found but also B3 (nicotinic acid) and B1 (thiamine). [184] Rhizopus oligosporus, a fungus in the family Mucoraceae, is widely used as a starter for homemade tempeh. Although R. oligosporus can prevent the growth of other microorganisms, it grows well with lactic acid bacteria (LAB). Lactobacillus plantarum. Therefore, the development of a soybean-based functional food by the co-inoculation of R. oligosporus and L. plantarum is a promising approach to increase the bioactivity of tempeh. A study found that tempeh, produced with both L. plantarum and R. oligosporus, might be a beneficial dietary supplement for individuals with type 2 diabetes and insulin resistance. [185] Tempeh is not just for people who don't eat meat because tempeh is so healthy, has no cholesterol, and is an excellent way to get B vitamins, fiber, calcium, iron, and other minerals. You can benefit from probiotics and isoflavone; chemicals called phytoestrogen have antioxidant and cancer-fighting properties. Therefore, tempeh is a healthy way to add to any diet.

14. Traditional Buttermilk

There are two main types of buttermilk: traditional and cultured. Cultured buttermilk found in American supermarkets does not have any probiotic benefits. Traditional buttermilk is a leftover liquid by-product made during the churning of butter. It is a famous fermented drink in India and other Middle Eastern countries. Buttermilk has a fresh, piquant taste imparted by lactic acid bacteria (LAB), which remains an integral part of buttermilk even after fermentation. [186]

15. Yogurt

is one of the best-known foods that contain probiotics. Two of the main starter cultures in yogurt are Lactobacillus bulgaricus and Streptococcus thermophilus. The function of the starter cultures is to ferment the lactose (milk sugar) to produce lactic acid. The increase in lactic acid decreases pH and causes the milk to clot or form the soft gel characteristic of yogurt. The fermentation of lactose also produces the flavor compounds characteristic of yogurt. Lactobacillus bulgaricus and Streptococcus thermophilus are the only 2 cultures required by law (CFR) to be present in yogurt. Other bacterial cultures, such as Lactobacillus acidophilus, Lactobacillus subsp. Casei, Bifidobacterium bifidum, Bifidobacterium lactis, and Lactobacillus rhamnosus may be added to yogurt as probiotic cultures. Probiotic cultures benefit human health by improving lactose digestion, gastrointestinal function and stimulating the immune system. [187] However, keep in mind that not all yogurt is equal. Some of them do not contain live probiotics. Sometimes, the live bacteria have been wiped out during processing. This is important to choose yogurt with active or live cultures.

Most people think yogurt is the best probiotic, but I would tell you that is not true if *you are looking for the best probiotic from dairy. In that case, kefir is your best choice because Kefir has a wide variety of microorganisms. It also contains beneficial yeasts such as Saccharomyces cerevisiae and Saccharomyces unisporus. Kefir offers more protein than yogurt and less sugar as a nutritional value.*

16. The bonus. Ice Cream.

Yes, you heard it right, and I'm not joking. The main constituents of ice cream are fat, milk solids-not-fat (skim-milk powder), sugar, a suitable stabilizer such as gelatin, egg, and flavoring. By now, you have a lot of information about probiotics. You can use kefir or yogurt and cultured whipping cream for the homemade ice cream. So, you get the benefit from probiotics while having a delicious ice cream. I will add the recipes as well.

You might have heard about go-gurt, and you think it is made from yogurt and has a good potential for probiotic sources. From A Review: Factors Influencing Probiotic Survival in Ice Cream report that "Dairy frozen desserts which are prepared from yogurt, may decrease the bio-availability of Lactobacillus acidophilus and Bifidobacterium species because of low pH <4.5 (Ravula and Shah, 1998b), while the incorporation of probiotic bacteria in non-fermentative ice cream does not create any problem because ice cream pH (6.6-6.5) is ideal for probiotics survival" [188] So now you know if you are going to have a cold dessert, just go ahead with ice cream but not go-gurt because it doesn't offer as much as most people think.

In conclusion

Thriving gut flora is excellent for your body and brain. The live microorganism promotes your health and helps enhance weight loss and keep the weight off whether you prefer dairy or non-dairy choices. All are excellent. Make sure you have varieties of them because it's more beneficial with the diversity of the gut microbiome. So, from now on, you can enjoy delicious food while feeding your gut microbiome. You know what they love. It's important to know what they hate, too. The next chapter will learn what food and activities cause gut dysbiosis.

TO-DO LIST

- Add at least 5 prebiotic foods to your meal each day.

- Add at least 1-3 probiotic foods to your meal each day.

- If you have great recipes or favorite probiotic food that you found from a store, e.g., yogurt, kimchi, or kefir. Please share with the community on Facebook.

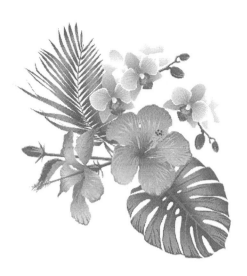

CHAPTER 6

GUT DYSBIOSIS

FOOD THAT KILLS YOUR GUT MICROBIOME

Previous chapter, you have learned what prebiotics and probiotics are. You can benefit from eating delicious food and creating a post-biotic for your gut. However, it's necessary to know what is not good for your gut ecosystem so that you will receive the maximum payoff from the gut microbiome. The microbiota contributes to energy extraction from food and the synthesis of vitamins and amino acids and helps create barriers against pathogens. Disruption of intestinal microbiota homeostasis—called dysbiosis—has been associated with inflammatory bowel disease (IBD), irritable bowel syndrome (IBS), celiac disease, food allergies, type 1 diabetes, type 2 diabetes, cancer, obesity, and cardiovascular disease. Although it is unclear whether dysbiosis is the cause or the result of these diseases, factors that contribute to the development and progression of many of these diseases influence the GIT microbiota. Dysbiosis can be caused by environmental factors that frequently come across in Western societies as follows; [189]

1. **Alcohol**

or ethanol is addictive, toxic, and can have harmful physical and mental effects when overconsumption—according to the record of World

Health Organization 2016, accounting for over 3 million deaths (5.3% of all deaths) worldwide and 132.6 million disability-adjusted life years (DALYs). Excessive alcohol consumption is a global healthcare problem with enormous social, economic, and clinical consequences. Excessive drinking over decades damages every organ in the body. However, the liver has the quickest and the greatest tissue damage from excessive alcohol because it is the main section of ethanol metabolism. [190]

Alcohol is related to an increase in the risk of both liver cirrhosis and pancreatitis, leading to about 637,000 digestive disease deaths and 23.3 million digestive disease DALYs in 2016. Within the burden of alcohol-attributable digestive diseases, alcohol-attributable liver cirrhosis caused 607,000 deaths and 22.2 million DALYs, while alcohol-attributable pancreatitis occurred in 30,000 deaths and 1.1 million DALYs. [191]

Chronic alcohol consumption in humans also causes bacterial overgrowth and dysbiosis. Heavy alcohol consumption will alter communication between the gut and liver, not only by increasing circulating alcohol and producing acetaldehyde, which can damage the liver at high concentrations but also by enabling harmful gut microbiota-derived molecules to leak into the circulation and inflict damage on both the intestinal wall and the liver. [192]

So, what is chronic alcohol consumption?

According to the "Dietary Guidelines for Americans 2020-2025," U.S. Department of Health and Human Services and U.S. Department of Agriculture, adults of legal drinking age can choose not to drink or to **drink in moderation** by limiting intake to 2 drinks or fewer in a day for men and 1 drink or less in a day for women when alcohol is consumed.

National Institute on Alcohol Abuse and Alcoholism (NIAAA) defines heavy drinking:

For men, consuming over 4 drinks on any day or over 14 drinks per week.

For women, consuming over 3 drinks on any day or over 7 drinks per week.

If you can limit your drink each time to one drink for women or 2 drinks for men, that would be ok. But unfortunately, most people can't stop just 1 or 2 drinks, or someone like me who goes for "all or nothing" would be better off; otherwise, you might go over the limit. One day my mother asked me why I had to drink? I drink only wine, so I told my mother that drinking wine is excellent for health. You know Mom is always right! However, I tried to prove to her from a scientific perspective which she might not know.

NOT ALL ALCOHOL IS BAD

So here is what I found from the studies. *"Influence of red wine polyphenols and ethanol on the gut microbiota ecology and biochemical biomarkers"* It's a comparison between red wine (Alcohol and polyphenols), dealcoholized red wine (no alcohol and polyphenols), and gin (alcohol and no polyphenols). They found that gin decreased the number of beneficial gut bacteria. Alcohol only is not good, so we can get this one out of the picture. Next, the daily consumption of red wine polyphenol for 4 weeks significantly increased the number of gut bacteria *(Enterococcus, Prevotella, Bacteroides, Bifidobacterium, Bacteroides uniformis). Eggerthella lenta, and Blautia coccoides-Eubacterium rectale groups.)* In the meantime, systolic and diastolic blood pressures and triglyceride, total cholesterol, HDL cholesterol, and C-reactive protein concentrations declined significantly. Changes in cholesterol and

C-reactive protein concentrations were linked to changes in the bifidobacteria number. The beneficial effect of daily red wine consumption in moderation on gut bacteria appears to be because of its polyphenol content. However, the concentrations of Bacteroides and Firmicutes decreased after the dealcoholized red wine period compared with the red wine period.

> *Sweet surprise*
>
> *They also found that red wine polyphenols can prevent harmful bacteria and help the growth of good bacteria, such as bifidobacteria, which could be supported in reducing CRP and cholesterol observed in our study, promoting health benefits in the host.* [193]

Another study showed that polyphenol from cocoa flavanols plus ethanol intake affected the growth of the Blautia coccoides–Eubacterium rectale group, Bifidobacterium, Eggerthella lenta, and Bacteroides uniformis. The last 2 microorganisms can degrade resveratrol into dihydro resveratrol, which has antiproliferative effects on human prostate cancer cells. [194] [195] Red wine is rich in a great variety of polyphenolic compounds with potential neuroprotective activities, such as Alzheimer's disease (AD). [196]

Wine polyphenols are divided into two categories: flavonoids and non-flavonoids. The flavonoids account for most of the polyphenolic components in red wine (>85%, ≥1 g/L) and contain compounds such as anthocyanins.

In conclusion, alcoholics have an altered colonic microbiome (dysbiosis). [197] However, red wine is exceptional because predominant red wine polyphenols, such as flavan-3-ol monomers and procyanidins, are related to antimicrobial activity. Red wine brings a unique and very diverse combination of phenolic structures, including flavonols, flavan-3-ols, and anthocyanins, among the flavonoid compounds, and hydroxybenzoic and hydroxycinnamic acids, phenolic alcohols, and stilbenes, among the non-flavonoids. Considering the influence of wine polyphenols on human microbiota is becoming widely recognized. Phenolic compounds present in red wine have shown antioxidant and anti-inflammatory properties, reduced insulin resistance and benefitted by reducing oxidative stress. As a result, a simple effect on reducing risk factors and the prevention of cardiovascular diseases has been observed.

The key is that drinking red wine daily in moderation will be the most beneficial for your health and the gut microbiome. Ok! So now it's my answer to my mother. This time I'm right!

2. Antibiotics

are powerful prescriptions used to treat infections and conditions caused by bacteria and pathogens, such as strep throat and urinary tract infection. The widespread use of antibiotics in the past 80 years has saved millions of human lives. They act by either killing bacteria or prohibiting them from multiplying. However, they kill both good and bad bacteria. Even a single antibiotic approach can lead to adverse changes in the balance and diversity of the gut flora.

Mounting evidence appears that antibiotics influence the function of the immune system, our ability to resist infection, and our capacity for processing food. Both human and animal studies have proved that even a one-time antibiotic treatment can lead to decreases in bacteria considered beneficial, such as bifidobacteria and Lactobacilli, as well as increases in potential pathogens such as Clostridium difficile and the yeast Candida albicans. In the short term, such shifts in microbiota can cause yeast infections and GI symptoms, including bloating, abdominal pain, and diarrhea, but recent work suggests the consequences may be much longer lasting and more serious.[198]

Antibiotics interfere with the interaction between the microbiome and immune system, resulting in immunological disorders; antibiotics also increase the host's susceptibility to pathogens. Antibiotic exposure during infancy has been found to increase the risk of overweight in preadolescence for boys. The risk of developing type 2 diabetes increases with repeated penicillins, macrolides, cephalosporins, and quinolones. [199]

Have you ever heard of *"antibiotic-resistant"*? According to *CDC's Antibiotic Resistance Threats in the United States, 2019 (2019 AR Threats Report)*, over 2.8 million antibiotic-resistant infections occur in the U.S. each year, and over 35,000 people die. In addition, 223,900 cases of Clostridium difficile (C. diff) occurred in 2017 and at least 12,800 people died. [200]

ANTIBIOTIC RESISTANCE IS A GLOBAL PUBLIC HEALTH CRISIS

Before the pandemic COVID-19, the CDC and WHO were always aware that antibiotic resistance is one of the biggest threats to global health, food security, and development. Antibiotic resistance is rising too high levels in all parts of the world that can affect anyone, any age, and any country.

> *Antibiotic resistance (AR) occurs when bacteria change in response to the use of these medicines.*
>
> *Antimicrobial Resistance (AMR) occurs when bacteria, viruses, fungi, and parasites change over time and no longer respond to medicines, making infections harder to treat and increasing the risk of disease spread, severe illness, and death.* [201]

In 2014, Lord Jim O'Neill and his team published a review commissioned by the United Kingdom government entitled, "Antimicrobial Resistance: Tackling a crisis for the health and wealth of nations." The study estimated that antimicrobial resistance (AMR) could cause 10 million deaths a year by 2050. [202]

Some facts that have contributed to this crisis include the over prescription of antibiotics, insufficient laboratory tests to identify an infection, and poor hygiene practices in hospitals. However, the most crucial factor that may lead to human drug resistance is the overuse of antibiotics in farming and agriculture. Of all antibiotics sold in the United States, 80% are sold for animal agriculture. Antibiotics apply to animals in feed to improve growth rates and prevent infections, and a practice projected to increase worldwide over the next 15 years. [203] Demand for animal protein for human consumption is rising globally at an unusual rate. Global consumption of antimicrobials in food animal production was estimated at 63,151 (±1,560) tons in 2010 and is projected to rise by 67%, to 105,596 (±3,605) tons, by 2030. [204] You know the equation of demand and supply.

The first antibiotic, Penicillin, was invented in the 1928s by Alexander Fleming. It has saved millions of lives in the past, especially during World War II. But nowadays, why do antibiotics become resistant? Antibiotics are excellent to use when you have a bacterial infection such as strep throat, pneumonia, urinary infection but not the common cold, flu, or athlete's foot. We misuse it, use it too much, and use it without caution. Antibiotics are miracle drugs that can work when we really need them. For example, surgery like heart surgery, joint replacement, cancer, or chemotherapy. But once it becomes resistant, now in the critical moment, we have nothing to save those lives.

Alexander Fleming warned, *"An ignorant man may under-dose himself... make them resistant, rendering penicillin ineffective in the future"* He knew from the beginning if you use too low a dose of penicillin or if you give an intermittent dose, the bacteria become resistant.

You might think that the Antibiotic resistance might happen only in the hospital, but it's all everywhere, from the household, your pets, farm, water, and on land. It's not only your health, but the community is one health because it can transmit to a person, from your pet to you and now the soil that we grow vegetables. Using antibiotics in animal husbandry in therapeutic and subtherapeutic doses creates selective pressure for antibiotic resistance genes (ARGs) in the animal's gut microbiome, which is then excreted in the feces. Therefore, manure application to agricultural land is a potential route for the transmission of antibiotic-resistant bacteria from livestock to crops, animals, and humans. The link between human health, animal health, plant health, and the environment is crucial.[205]

A recent publication in the National Center for Biotechnology Information (NCBI) and U.S. National Institutes of Health's National Library of Medicine in May 2021 *"Antimicrobial Residues in Food from Animal Origin—A Review of the Literature Focusing on Products Collected in Stores and Markets Worldwide,"* Here is a summary of this publishing "The extensive use of antibiotics leads to antibiotic residues in consumed foods. The primary use of antibiotics in animals is to treat and prevent diseases and growth promotion. However, the residues and their breakdown products have several side effects on the human body and, in a broader sense, on the environment. A wide range of antibiotics has been found in the following products: milk, eggs, poultry, beef, pork, seafood, fish, and lamb. The most common prescriptions for people are penicillins, macrolides, and fluoroquinolones.

In contrast, tetracyclines and sulfonamides are most commonly used in animal breeding. These substances' residues and degradation products have many undesirable side effects on the human body. It influences the immune system, damages the kidneys (gentamicin), increases the frequency of mutations, can damage the liver, damages the bone marrow (chloramphenicol), and affects the human reproductive organs. Carcinogenic effects have been found with antibiotics such as sulfamethazine, oxytetracycline, and furazolidone. Maximum residue limits of antibiotics regarding food help protect consumers, but there are no guarantees that animal products exceeding the limits will not come onto the market and be consumed by people. Even if the maximum residue limits for antibiotics in foods of animal origin are not exceeded, they can still lead to problems in the long term. For example, nitrofurazone is an antibiotic with carcinogenic properties. It can affect the DNA of cells and result in genetic toxicity that can cause cancer. This antibiotic has been found, especially in shrimps but also in aquaculture catfish. A particular challenge, in this case, is that this molecule is not so easy to detect. The right technology and the associated equipment are required to provide reliable evidence. Especially in underdeveloped countries regarding food safety, so nitrofurazone often goes undetected, and thus, contaminated products are also distributed on the world market and ultimately consumed." [206]

HOW TO STOP ANTIBIOTIC RESISTANCE AND ANTIMICROBIAL RESISTANCE

1. **Stop consuming beef, pork, chicken, egg, milk, fish, seafood, and lamb. If there is less demand, then there will be less supply. If you can't stop eating this type of food, then chose the next one.**

2. **Consuming animal products with no antibiotic use only.**

How do you know about it?

According to Consumer Reports' Guide to Food Label Seals & Claims.

1. **Organic means:**

- Minimal pesticide residues.

- Animals raised without antibiotics or added hormones.

- No genetically modified (or engineered) organisms (GMOs).

- Strong standards, backed by federal law.

- Annual on-farm inspections are required.

Not giving antibiotics to animals raised for meat, poultry, dairy, and eggs is one of the many requirements that food producers must meet to use the Department of Agriculture's organic seal on their products.

One exception: Chickens and turkeys can be given antibiotics in the hatchery while the chick is still in the egg and on its first day of life. But if you also see a "raised without antibiotics" claim on a chicken or turkey product besides the USDA organic label, it means antibiotics were not used at any point, even in the hatcheries.

For eggs: The chickens must be raised organically from the age of 2 days; have much the same rights to a safe, healthy environment as cattle do; and have the same rules against antibiotic use. They have to be fed only organic feed that isn't genetically modified and is grown without synthetic pesticides or GMOs. However, organic doesn't mean the chickens are roaming free outdoors, but they must have outdoor access. 207

For seafood and fish: Choose wild-caught fish and seafood but not farm-raised, especially shrimps, catfish, and tilapia which came from developing countries such as India, Vietnam, China, and Thailand. There is a lot of documentation that found fish and seafood from those countries have antimicrobial residues and antibiotics residues in a greater amount. [208] [209] [210] [211] [212] It's better to choose local shrimp rather than importing from Asia. You can watch more videos from YouTube for your education and information about seafood from Asia such as;

- Testing shrimp for antibiotic-resistant bacteria (Marketplace) by CBC NEWS on Mar 15, 2019,

- What should we think about Shrimp by Doctor OZ on Nov 11, 2019,

- The dirty business with the shrimps by Free high-quality documentaries on Aug 23, 2019.

2. **Raised Without Antibiotics**

This and related phrases, such as "no antibiotics ever" and "never given antibiotics," mean no antibiotics of any kind were used in the raising of that animal. Producers send documentation to the USDA to support their claim, but there are no inspections. However, if the package also sports a USDA Process Verified seal, it means that USDA inspectors have visited the farm to confirm that antibiotics were not used.

There are several companies that produce or serve meat raised without antibiotics. For example, Chipotle and Panera both serve beef and chicken raised without antibiotics and have third parties conduct at least some audits of their practices. Bell & Evans falls into this category, as do Perdue and Tyson. Progresso uses no-antibiotics chicken in all its chicken soup varieties. Applegate Farms and Coleman Natural produce no-antibiotics, poultry, beef, and pork.

3. **No Medically Important Antibiotics**

This means antibiotics used to treat people—such as amoxicillin, erythromycin, and tetracycline—have never been given to the animals.

However, "no medically important antibiotics" doesn't mean "no antibiotics." And even antibiotics that aren't medically important may lead to resistance to other antibiotics.

4. No Critically Important Antibiotics

This means the company has stopped using only some of the medically important antibiotics used to treat people.

And with poultry, a "no critically important antibiotics" claim doesn't translate to meaningful change in antibiotic use.

5. No Growth-Promoting Antibiotics

The "no growth-promoting antibiotics" label means no antibiotics were fed to the animal to speed up growth. However, in the fine print on its label that antibiotics can be used for disease prevention, consumers may misinterpret this claim.

"To preserve antibiotic effectiveness for people, the drugs should be used only when animals are sick."

6. One Health Certified

One Health Certified is a label developed by meat and poultry industry experts. It is used only on chicken and turkey meat packages sold in supermarkets such as Aldi and BJ's Wholesale Club. It's meant to show a company's commitment to animal welfare, environmental issues, and responsible antibiotic use.

Restrictions on the use of antibiotics are minimal, and meat from animals treated with antibiotics can be sold with the One Health Certified label. In addition, under the label's Life Cycle Assessment requirement, producers must measure their carbon footprint but don't have to take any action to reduce it. [213]

3. The recommendation from WHO [214]

To prevent and control the spread of antibiotic resistance, individuals can:

- Only use antibiotics when prescribed by a certified health professional.

- Never demand antibiotics if your health worker says you don't need them.

- Always follow your health worker's advice when using antibiotics.

- Never share or use leftover antibiotics.

- Prevent infections by regularly washing hands, preparing food hygienically, avoiding close contact with sick people, practicing safer sex, and keeping vaccinations up to date.

- Prepare food hygienically, following the WHO Five Keys to Safer Food (keep clean, separate raw and cooked, cook thoroughly, keep food at safe temperatures, use safe water and raw materials) and choose foods that have been produced without the use of antibiotics for growth promotion or disease prevention in healthy animals.

3. Artificial sweeteners

Recently, you saw more sugar-free foods in the market because people prefer to consume low-calorie content and the health matters about products with high sugar content. Sweeteners that are several hundred thousand times sweeter than sugar (or sucrose) are being consumed as sugar substitutes. Although nonnutritive sweeteners (NNSs) are considered safe and well-tolerated, their effects on glucose intolerance, the activation of sweet taste receptors, and alterations to the composition of the intestinal microbiota are controversial.

I have done deep research on this subject for you. Sweeteners have 2 types: Nonnutritive sweeteners and nutritive sweeteners.

1. Nonnutritive sweeteners (NNSs) have 2 types, first, *synthetic sweeteners* (such as; acesulfame K, aspartame, cyclamate, saccharin, neotame, advantame, and sucralose) and second, *natural sweeteners* (NSs; thaumatin, steviol glycosides, monellin, neohesperidin dihydrochalcone, Luo Han Guo fruit extracts, and glycyrrhizin)

2. Nutritive sweeteners (polyols or sugar alcohols)

To date, *the FDA has approved 6 high-intensity artificial sweeteners for foods and drinks: acesulfame potassium (acesulfame K), aspartame, neotame, saccharin, sucralose, and advantame.* In addition, *3 NNSs of natural origin—steviol glycosides, thaumatin, and Luo Han Guo fruit extracts (aka monk fruit extracts)—have been approved by the FDA.* The European Union (EU), the European Food Safety Authority (EFSA) has approved 11 NNSs for human consumption: acesulfame K (E-950), advantame (E-969), aspartame (E-951), aspartame-acesulfame salt (E-962), cyclamic acid and its sodium and calcium salts (E-952), neo hesperidin dihydrochalcone (E-959), neotame (E-961), saccharin (E-954), steviol glycosides (E-960, including 10 different glycosides), sucralose (E-955), and thaumatin (E-957).

WHICH SWEETENERS ARE GOOD, AND WHICH ONE IS BAD?

Food-use–approved polyols are low-calorie carbohydrates with a sweet taste used, volume-for-volume, as a substitute for sucrose and other free sugars. They include erythritol, hydrogenated starch hydrolysates (sometimes listed as maltitol syrup, hydrogenated glucose syrup, polyglycitol, polyglucitol, or HSH), isomalt, lactitol, maltitol, mannitol, sorbitol, and xylitol. In the United States, the FDA classifies some polyols as Recognized As Safe (GRAS), whereas others are approved food additives. [215]

1. Acesulfame K

is 200 times sweeter than sugar and has been used in many foods in the United States, such as baked goods, candies, frozen desserts, beverages, and dessert mixes. Acesulfame potassium brand names include Sunett® and Sweet One®. According to the FDA, the acceptable daily intake (or ADI) has been set at 15 milligrams per kilogram (mg/kg) of body weight. Acesulfame K is not metabolized or stored in the body. After it is consumed, it's rapidly absorbed but then quickly excreted from the body via urine without being changed. This is one reason FDA and many health authorities in many countries have approved its use in the food supply. However, some research mentioned that Acesulfame K decreases glucose fermentation by the cecal microbiota in Cara rats, suggesting that sweeteners might affect glucose transport systems. Therefore, it may lead to harmful changes in human metabolism by disrupting glucose regulation. It affects the gut microbiome and body weight gain in mice. [216]

2. Aspartame

Aspartame is ~200 times sweeter than sugar. The ADI for aspartame is 40 mg/kg of body weight. Aspartame is incorporated into over 6000 products, including soft drinks, dessert mixes, frozen desserts and yogurt, chewable multivitamins, and breakfast cereals and it is sold under brand names such as Equal, NutraSweet. A 400-mg dose of aspartame did not affect the peak insulin concentrations in subjects with or without diabetes but caused a decrease in plasma glucose concentrations. From reading several pieces of research, I have concluded that aspartame is the worst choice for sweeteners. It affects every organ of the body even though it is less than 40 mg/kg of body weight.

Check it out for every part of your body.

- *It affected blood either more or less than at safe doses (40 mg/kg body weight). It Impaired delivery of oxygen to the tissues by red blood cells, red blood cell aging, altered neutrophil function, decreased T-cell proliferation, platelet hyperactivity, and hyperaggregability, upregulation of proinflammatory signaling.*

- *It affected the brain either more or less than at safe doses (40 mg/kg body weight). It impaired neurobehavioral parameters (learning and memory), dysfunction of neuronal cells, disruption of the blood-brain barrier, upregulation of neuroinflammation, which may start neurotrophic effects.*

- *It affected the liver either more or less than at safe doses (40 mg/kg body weight). It has been shown to impair the antioxidant status of the liver, which may lead to hepatocellular injury. During oxidative stress, the balance between ROS and antioxidants shifts toward increased production of the former, affecting the energetic and regenerative processes, resulting in hepatic damage (or liver failure).*

- *Kidney. Oxidative stress may lead to kidney injury. Both higher dosages and safe dosages of aspartame may induce oxidative stress in the kidneys of rats. It was suggested that oxidative stress may contribute to the progression of kidney fibrosis in the kidney, and chronic kidney disease may be associated with inflammation and upregulated inflammatory cytokines.*

- *Heart (including cardiometabolic effects), Aspartame may lead to oxidative stress in cardiac tissue and has been shown to impair cardiac function, resulting in reduced heart rate variability, sympathetic dominance, and loss of vagal tone. Losing a protective vagal tone would explain the increased susceptibility to cardiovascular disease. The toxic effect of aspartame may also induce structural changes in the muscular layer of the heart (the myocardium) that manifest as compensatory hypertrophy of myocytes, which is clinically observed as heart failure.*

- *The immune system, the oxidant/antioxidant balance, is critical for immune cell function. Aspartame may act as a chemical stressor and induce oxidative stress by disturbing the oxidant/antioxidant balance, which may alter the ability of the immune system to maintain homeostasis, as observed in an animal model. This oxidant/antioxidant imbalance may lead to variations in serum cytokine levels and to alterations in both cellular and humoral immunity.*

- *The gut microbiota, aspartame, may influence gut metabolism by changing the host metabolic phenotype, affecting the gut microbiota. Changes in the gut microbiota may interfere with the physiological responses that control homeostasis, alter the intestinal environment, trigger inflammatory processes associated with metabolic disorders, or disrupt sweet-taste* receptors in the gut that can affect glucose absorptive capacity and glucose homeostasis. [217] [218] [219]

Sweet surprise

Do you know what type of sweetener Coca-Cola uses in its product?

The answer is aspartame.

What Coca-Cola products contain aspartame? 13

❖ Coke Zero Sugar

❖ Diet Barq's

❖ Diet Coke

❖ Diet Coke Feisty Cherry

❖ Fanta Zero

❖ Fresca

❖ Gold Peak Diet Tea

❖ Mello Yello Zero

❖ Minute Maid Light

❖ Pibb Zero

❖ Seagram's Diet Ginger Ale

❖ Sprite Zero

❖ TaB

Do your popular sodas contain aspartame?

a. Coca-Cola

---

13 *What is aspartame?* (n.d.). The Coca-Cola Company. https://www.coca-colacompany.com/faqs/what-is-aspartame

No. Coca-Cola Classic taste is not sweetened with aspartame. Depending on where you are in the world, Coca-Cola uses either high fructose corn syrup or cane sugar.

b. Coke Zero

Yes. Coke Zero Sugar in the bottles and cans with a blend of aspartame and acesulfame potassium (or Ace-K).

c. Diet Coke

Yes. Diet Coke in the bottles and cans is sweetened with aspartame. Diet Coke is also offered sweetened with SPLENDA®.

d. Sprite

No, but Sprite Zero in the US is sweetened with a blend of aspartame and Ace-K.

3. Saccharin

Saccharin, known as the first chemically produced artificial sweetener, has been sold as Sweet 'N Low. A range of food and beverages are sweetened by saccharin, which is safe despite controversial debate about its potential cancer and other health risks. Its ADI is the lowest of all the intensive sweeteners (5 mg/kg body weight).

Saccharin may induce oxidative stress on the liver cells through lowering catalase activity and the total antioxidant concentration (TAC) in plasma. It was shown that saccharin affects both liver and kidney tissue and alters biochemical markers, not only at high doses but also at low doses in rats. [220] As for cancer and toxicity are arguable because the studies in animals showed it causes cancer, but in human studies, some found the link between bladder cancer risk in humans, but most studies found no association between saccharin and cancer. However, long-term consumption increases the risk of obesity and diabetes since consumption of large amounts of saccharin (135 mg) may cause hypoglycemia (low blood sugar), reduced hyperinsulinemia (the amount of insulin in the blood is higher than considered normal amongst people without diabetes), and decreased insulin resistance in animal studies. [221]

As for gut microbiota, there were major shifts in microbial composition, making a significant influence on driving bacterial community dynamics.

4. Sucralose

Sucralose, sold as Splenda has become one of the most popular artificial sweeteners in the United States. Although made from sugar, it's not a natural product. By using a chemical process, sucralose becomes 400 to 700 times sweeter than sugar. Its ADI is 5 mg/kg body weight. In 1999, the U.S. Food and Drug Administration (FDA) authorized sucralose as safe for human consumption. However, there are conflicting investigations on the safety of sucralose. Some of the potential negative effects of sucralose include increased blood glucose levels and insulin levels while decreasing insulin sensitivity [222] [223] [224] and this could affect everyone, especially those who want to lose weight and those with diabetes. Sucralose has a big impact by inhibiting the growth of beneficial bacteria in the GI tract and various environmental microbes. [225] [226] [227]

5. Steviol glycosides

or known as Stevia, is a non-nutritive natural sweetener extracted from the Stevia rebaudiana plant which is native to Paraguay, Brazil, and Argentina, where it has been used by indigenous people for centuries in medicines and to sweeten drinks such as maté, a green herbal tea. The plant was first brought to the attention of the rest of the world by the botanist Moises Santiago Bertoni in 1887, who learned of its properties from the Paraguayan Indians. The chemical characterization of the plant's natural constituents known as steviol glycosides, which handle its distinct sweet taste, was not identified until 1931 when 2 French chemists, Bridel and Lavielle, isolated stevioside a primary steviol glycoside from stevia leaves. In the 1990s, stevia extract was available in the United States as a dietary supplement in health food stores. It is 50–350 times sweeter than table sugar. Its ADI is 4 mg/kg body weight. It doesn't cause cancer and isn't associated with any reproductive/developmental toxicity. Studies observed no significant impact on blood glucose in healthy or diabetic individuals and also suggested that steviol glycosides may have a positive effect on β cell function in subjects with type 2 diabetes. However, the current studies show that steviol glycosides have minimal impact on the gut microbiota. Bacteroides are the most efficient group of bacteria at hydrolyzing stevioside. Other bacterial groups, such as lactobacilli, bifidobacteria, Clostridium, coliforms, and enterococci species, weren't able to hydrolyze and use steviol glycosides as a usable substrate. So, it has a limitation of microbiota, especially the beneficial one. [228] However, one of the genius things about plants. The roots of Stevia contain inulin and fructans, functional food ingredients that positively affect human health and improve the growth of select microbial strains (bifidobacteria and lactobacilli) that are important for gut health. [229] [230]

> *Sweet surprise*
>
> *Stevia can help you look leaner by dropping water weight.*
>
> *How? Because it can increase sodium excretion and cause the kidney to expel the sodium. It's a cool trick, right?* [231]

6. Glycyrrhizin (Licorice)

Glycyrrhizin comes from the roots and rhizomes of Glycyrrhiza glabra (licorice). It is 30–200 times sweeter than sugar and is safe if <100 mg/d is ingested. Glycyrrhizin is anti-cancer, anti-inflammatory, antioxidant, antiviral, and prevents damage to the liver. [232] [233] However, it has potential hypertensive effects and an intense aftertaste.

> ### Sweet surprise
>
> *Recent studies found glycyrrhizin should be assessed for treatment of severe acute respiratory syndrome coronavirus (SARS-CoV)-2, which causes COVID-19.* [234] [235] [236]

In the gut, licorice is de-glycosylated to glycyrrhizic acid (the major product). These glycyrrhizin metabolites (especially 18β-glycyrrhetinic acid) are the best weapon to kill cancer cells such as; tumor cells. They exert potent inhibitory effects on rotavirus infection (rotavirus is a virus that causes gastroenteritis. Symptoms include severe diarrhea, vomiting, fever, and dehydration). [237]

7. Luo Han Guo fruit extracts (aka monk fruit extracts)

During the last decade, dried fruits of Siraitia grosvenorii Swingle fruit extract (SGFE), also known as Luo Han Guo or monk fruit, have turned into a popular natural sweetener. Luo Han Guo extracts, which are promoted as non-caloric natural sweeteners, are now incorporated into dietary supplements, protein powder, and soft drinks.

Luo Han Guo is native to the southern parts of China, mainly the Guangxi Province, and it has been used in herbal medicines such as treating coughs, sore throat, and excessive phlegm for centuries. The compounds that give ripe monk fruit its sweetness are called mogrosides. Mogrosides are not absorbed in the upper gastrointestinal tract and do not add any calories to your diet. When they enter the colon, gut microbes cleave off the glucose molecules and use them as an energy source. [238] [239] [240]

Monk fruit extract contains varying levels of mogrosides, which are 150 to 200 times sweeter than sugar. It's safe to use as a sweetener. Monk fruit sweeteners have been recognized as safe (GRAS) by the FDA since 2010 and not specified for ADI. (A numerical ADI may not be deemed necessary for several reasons, including evidence of the ingredient's safety at levels well above the amounts needed to achieve the desired effect (e.g., as a sweetener) in food.)

This wonderful, sweet thing not only contains zero calories, zero carbohydrates, and zero sugars, but it's also a source of antioxidants. It prevents liver damage, improves immune function and phlegm-relieving, and has anti-inflammatory, anti-microbial, anti-hyperglycemic, antitussive, anticancer, anti-fatigue , and anti-hyperlipidemic effects. *(Hyperlipidemia is elevated levels of any or all lipids (fats, cholesterol, or triglycerides) or lipoproteins in the blood.)* [241] [242] [243] [244]

8. Thaumatin

Thaumatin is a sweet protein isolated from the fruit of Thaumatococcus daniellii Benth (aka Katemfe), a plant native to tropical West Africa. Thaumatin is 100,000 times sweeter than sugar and licorice after-taste. It is safe for use as a sweetener with no ADI specified, which means it can be used according to GMP (Good manufacturing practice). Thaumatin has been approved as a sweetener in the European Union, Israel, and Japan. However, it has not been approved as a sweetener in the USA but has a GRAS status as a flavor enhancer. Interestingly, this sweet fruit has protein but not carbohydrates like other sweet fruit. So, after digestion, it has 4 kcal/g as protein. [245]

Next is nutritive sweeteners.

Polyhydric sugar alcohols (sugar alcohols, polyols) are low digestible carbohydrates in fruits, vegetables, mushrooms, and human organisms. The most important and most commonly used polyols in food products are sorbitol, xylitol, maltitol, mannitol, erythritol, isomalt, and lactitol. They are mainly produced from corresponding sugars by catalytic hydrogenation; however, mannitol can be extracted from seaweed, while erythritol is got in fermentative processes led by osmophilic yeasts, such as Moniliella pollinis or Trichosporonoides megachiliensis. Polyols' sweetness varies from 25% to 100% as compared with table sugar. Thus, they are often used in combination with other sweeteners to achieve the desired flavor and level of sweetness. They are used volume-for-volume like sugar and are called bulk sweeteners. Similarly, to carbohydrates, they also play a role in retaining moisture and texture and product preservation. Sugar alcohol's glycemic index is much smaller than sugars. Thus, they are used to sweeten food products for people with diabetes. The bacteria in the mouth do not break them down, so they do not lead to dental cavities, and it's the perfect ingredient for chewing gum. In addition, they can be used as probiotics and anti-caries agents. The FDA, Codex Alimentarius, and EFSA have approved 8 different polyols— erythritol, hydrogenated starch hydrolysates, isomalt, lactitol, maltitol, mannitol, sorbitol, and xylitol—for use as bulk sweeteners in human foods.

- **Erythritol** occurs in nature and foods such as wine, beer, mushrooms, pears, grapes, and soy sauce. It is produced from glucose by an osmophilic yeast and, by separation and purification, yields a crystalline product with a purity of 99%. Erythritol is rapidly absorbed in the small intestine and excreted in the urine. It does not affect plasma glucose, insulin concentrations, or gut microbiota. It is considered a safe additive that doesn't cause cancer, has no toxicity, and is a harmful substance that affects the reproductive system.[246] You can see it with natural sweeteners such as stevia extract (Truvia brand) and monk fruit extract (Lakanto brand, whole earth brand).

- **Isomalt** is considered a prebiotic carbohydrate contributing to a healthy luminal colonic mucosal environment. It was reported that isomalt fermented in the gut increased bifidobacteria in vitro. Several bifidobacteria strains could metabolize the isomalt and generated high butyrate concentrations.[247]

- **Lactitol** is a non–naturally occurring sugar alcohol obtained by the hydrogenation of lactose. Lactitol is hardly absorbed in the small intestine (only in 2% by passive diffusion) and mainly is fermented in the large intestine, where it is transformed into biomass, short-chain fatty acids, carbon dioxide, a small amount of hydrogen, and organic acids. Lactitol acts as a prebiotic, stimulating Lactobacilli and Bifidobacteria growth.[248]

- **Maltitol** is obtained by the hydrolysis, reduction, and hydrogenation of starch, resulting in a sweetener with ~90% sweetening capacity. It doesn't cause cancer. *Maltitol is not completely digested and results in a slower rise in blood sugar and insulin levels.* It is fermented in the colon, and some people experience stomach pains and gas. One study in 2010 showed the numbers of fecal bifidobacteria, lactobacilli, and SCFAs significantly increased after the ingestion of maltitol compared with the ingestion of sugar.[249]

- **Mannitol** is an occurring six-carbon sugar alcohol that has wide applications in the food and pharmaceutical industry such as dental hygiene products, drug fillers, and as a diuretic in intravenous fluids because of its many properties, being a natural sweetener with low metabolism and no glycemic index. [250] To my knowledge, no data on the effects of mannitol on the gut microbiota is available.

- **Sorbitol**, also known as d-glucitol, is found in apples, pears, peaches, apricots, and some vegetables. It's safe for healthy individuals, but it can be of concern for patients with IBS, and there are reports of laxative effects when consumed in high doses. Most healthy individuals tolerate ~10 g sorbitol/d with only mild gastrointestinal discomfort, such as flatulence or bloating. However, there is not enough data to date to determine the effects of sorbitol on gut microbiota.

- **Xylitol**, a five-carbon polyol, obtained by the hydrogenation of d-xylose is found in fruits, berries, vegetables, oats, and mushrooms and the human body also produces a small percentage. Besides sugar-free candies and chewing gums, xylitol is widely used in various pharmaceutical products. Xylitol was first synthesized in 1891 and is ~95% as sweet as sugar. The effects of the intake of xylitol on the composition of gut microbiota are incredible. Xylitol ingestion shifted the rodent fecal microbiome population from Gram-negative to Gram-positive bacteria. The study showed the combination of lactobacilli (probiotic), and xylitol (prebiotic) had a protective effect against C. difficile infection as well. [251] [252]

In Conclusion

As you can see, the non-nutritive sweeteners (NNSs) first type, synthetic sweeteners (acesulfame potassium, aspartame, neotame, saccharin, sucralose, and advantame.) are harmful to your body and your gut microbiome. Even though the FDA is approved, you can see the evidence from research and studies that they might contribute to the development of metabolic derangements that lead to obesity, type 2 diabetes, cardiovascular disease, and the risk of cancer.

Second, the natural sweeteners (thaumatin, stevia, monk fruit extracts, and licorice) are safe for your body, and your gut, except stevia extracts, which may affect gut microbiota composition.

Last, nutritive sweeteners (polyols or sugar alcohols) even though all the names sound artificial, but they are not, and we call them sugar alcohols, but it's not alcohol. You will notice they are a mixture of stevia extract products or monk fruit extract products and in products for diabetes. So now you learn they are safe to consume, and it's terrific for your gut and several polyols, including isomalt and maltitol, increase bifidobacteria quantities in healthy individuals, and these polyols may have prebiotic actions. Only caution they might create gas or bloating since they reach the colon, especially in patients with inflammatory bowel disease. Another note for glycemic index: all of them are low glycemic index except that the maltitol glycemic index is 3, which may raise your blood sugar level.

4. Diet high in sugar

From chapter 1, you learn the daily sugar limit is 6 tsp (25 g) for women and 9 tsp (38 g) for men. You go over the limit if you eat food from the package and manufactured foods. High sugars and poor plant-derived fibers are associated with an increased risk of metabolic and cardiovascular diseases and chronic inflammation.

Recent studies have shown that a high intake of sugars increases the relative affluence of Proteobacteria (gram-negative) in the gut, while together decreasing the abundance of Bacteroides (Bacteroides dominates in slimmer people) which can mitigate the effects of endotoxin, as well as support gut barrier function. Therefore, a high sugar intake may overwhelm the balance of microbiota to have developed pro-inflammatory properties and decrease the capacity to regulate epithelial integrity and decreased immune-regulatory functions. High levels of glucose or fructose in the diet regulate the gut microbiota and increase intestinal permeability, which precedes the development of metabolic endotoxemia, inflammation, and fat accumulation, leading to fatty liver disease and normal-weight obesity. 253

(Normal-weight obesity syndrome is characterized by excess body fat in individuals with adequate body mass index. This condition increases the risk of cardiovascular morbidity and mortality and other conditions associated with chronic diseases, such as insulin resistance, hypertension, and dyslipidemia, aka an abnormal level of cholesterol and other lipids). 254 255

5. Diet high in fat

High-fat diets (HFDs) are associated with obesity. It impacts gut microbiota and metabolic disorders. It induces gut microbiome dysbiosis and colonic inflammation, and it leads to gastrointestinal disease occurrence and development. A diet that is high in fat, especially high in saturated and trans-fat, can create dysbiosis of intestinal flora composition and contribute to a variety of gastrointestinal and systemic diseases such as Inflammatory bowel diseases (IBD), irritable bowel syndrome (IBS), colorectal cancer, and Nonalcoholic fatty liver disease. 256 257

Most saturated fat is from animal fat. You should avoid or use sparing the following.

- Fatty cuts from beef, pork, lamb, and that includes bacon.

- Dark skin from poultry, fat, and skin.

- High-fat dairy foods (butter, whole milk, cheese, sour cream)

- Lard. (So many studies show it can cause liver damage, fatty liver, cause thyroid dysfunction, cause obesity, impaired glucose tolerance, lower fasting insulin levels, lower counts of enteroendocrine cells (or gut endocrine cells), and elevated cholesterol level, LDL, triglyceride and non-HDL.[258] [259] [260] [261] [262]

Saturated fat coconut oil is exceptional because it is a saturated oil (about 90%), but 63.3% of its total fatty acid composition is a medium-chain fatty acid (MCFA). Your body is absorbed MCFA through the small intestines. They do not need pancreatic lipase for digestion then travel through the portal vein directly to the liver where they are immediately converted into energy rather than being stored as fat, unlike long-chain fatty acids (LCFA) are often stored as fat, and if an excess is consumed, it can increase the risk of health problems like obesity and heart disease. Long-chain fatty acids such as animal fats, dairy fat, all vegetable oil, avocado, and olive oil are included.

MCFAs in coconut oil can help stimulate your body's metabolism, leading to weight loss.[263] However, use it in moderation because coconut oil is not 100% MCFAs, unlike MCT oil.

WHAT'S THE DIFFERENCE BETWEEN COCONUT OIL AND MCT OIL?

MCT (Medium-chain triglyceride) has a lot of health benefits such as fat loss, brain health, antimicrobial properties, helps protect your heart, helps to manage blood sugar, aids Alzheimer's disease, epilepsy, and autism. [264] MCT is hydrolyzed both faster and more extensively during digestion. Most of the remaining non-hydrolyzed MCT are absorbed by intestinal cells. So, you won't store fat from MCT oil. *The term medium-chain triglyceride (MCT) is used to refer to two main types of triglycerides: a synthetic triglyceride mixture containing C8 and C10 (that is, commercial MCT oil)* and natural triglycerides which contain only C6 to C12. "MCT oil" has the following approximate composition:

C6: 1-2%, C8: 65-75%, C10: 25-35%, C12: 2% (max.)

> *Medium-chain fatty acids (MCFAs) have chains of 6-12 carbon atoms. The MCFAs in this group are C6 (caproic acid), C10 (capric acid), C8 (caprylic acid), and C12 (lauric acid).*
>
> *Long-chain fatty acids (LCFAs) have chains of 14-22 carbon atoms. The long chain saturated fatty acids found in coconut oil are C14 (myristic acid), C16 (palmitic acid), and C18 (stearic acid).*

Coconut oil has MCFA 63.3% and LCFA 30.8%. It has the following approximate composition; [265]

C6 (caproic): 0.4%, C8 (caprylic): 7.3%, C10 (capric): 6.5%, C12 (lauric): 49.2% , C14 (myristic): 18.9%, C16 (palmitic) 8.9% , C18 (stearic) 3.0%, C18:1 (oleic) 7.5%, C18:2 (linoleic) 1.8%, C18:3 (linolenic) 0.1%

So now you can see the coconut oil is not 100% MCFA, unlike MCT oil. You can use MCT oil in your coffee or smoothie, but you can't cook with it. So, coconut is perfect for cooking.

Trans fat increases the risk of heart disease and type 2 diabetes.

Trans fat is short for trans fatty acids. You should avoid this type of fat because it can raise LDL, also known as bad cholesterol, and lower your HDL, known as "good" cholesterol. It can increase your risk of developing heart disease and stroke and is also associated with a higher risk of developing type 2 diabetes.

There are two types of trans fats discovered in foods: occurring and artificial trans fats. Naturally occurring trans fats are presented in the gut of some animals, and foods created from these animals (for example, meat and milk products) may have small portions of these fats.

Artificial trans fats (or trans fatty acids) are made in an industrial process that adds hydrogen to liquid vegetable oils to prepare them more stable. [266] *The primary dietary source for trans fats in processed food is "partially hydrogenated oils." You might find trans-fat* in

- Processed foods (crackers, microwave popcorn, frozen pizza)
- Fried foods (deep-fried fast doughnuts)
- Margarine
- Vegetable shortening
- Vegetable oil
- Bakery products (cakes, cookies, pastries)
- Non-Dairy Coffee Creamers

In addition, you have heard about "heating vegetable oils are loaded with polyunsaturated fats that are fragile and oxidize in heat"? **Yes, heating can turn vegetable oil to be trans-fat.**

From the Acta Scientific Nutritional Health journal in 2018, "Evaluation of Chemical and Physical Changes in Different Commercial

Oils during Heating," **this study reveals that smoke points do not predict oil performance when heated. Oxidative stability and UV coefficients are better predictors when combined with the total level of PUFAs.** Of all the oils tested (Extra Virgin Olive Oil, Virgin Olive Oil, Olive Oil, Canola Oil, Rice Bran Oil, Grapeseed Oil, Coconut Oil, Peanut Oil, Sunflower Oil, and Avocado Oil), Extra virgin olive oil (EVOO) was the oil that produced the lowest level of polar compounds after being heated followed by coconut oil. [267]

WHICH OILS ARE GOOD FOR YOU?

So, from now on, you know the only 2 oils that you will bring home are extra virgin olive oil and unrefined coconut oil. The high content of antioxidant polyphenols (hydroxytyrosol, oleuropein) makes extra virgin olive oil stable and resistant to oxidation and minimizes cancer risk. [268] Coconut oil has a significant benefit for cardiovascular and other health benefits since it is rich in lauric acid. The new study in 2021 demonstrated that replacement of PUFA-rich oils with coconut oil significantly increased HDL (good cholesterol) but not LDL (bad cholesterol).[269]

A recent medical publication in 2021 mentioned that "according to 2020 statistics, 1,806,590 new cancer cases and 606,520 cancer deaths occurred in the United States, with gastrointestinal cancer being one of the leading causes of death. Colorectal cancer (CRC) is the most diagnosed and fatal gastrointestinal cancer. Pancreatic cancer is the second, with a five-year survival rate of only 9% in America. These are followed by liver, stomach, and esophageal cancers. Obesity is a risk factor for gastrointestinal cancer, and the primary cause of obesity is a high-fat diet (HFD). High-fat diets can cause metabolic reprogramming of multiple organs and tissues of the human body, with alterations in the content of various regulatory factors. It mainly acts on tumor cells themselves, nearby tissues, and the tumor microenvironment. [270] HFDs had higher growth and metabolic activity and increased expression of pro-inflammatory and tumorigenic factors such as leptin, IGFBP, FGF-α in their adipose tissue, in contrast to decreased anti-inflammatory and growth inhibition molecules. Clinical, epidemiological studies found that "meat and fat" cause esophagus cancer. [271]

IS THE KETO DIET GOOD FOR YOU AND YOUR GUT?

A study in 2020 regarding high-fat ketogenic diets (KDs) and gut microbiome for 8 weeks showed KDs alter the human and mouse gut microbiota in a manner distinct from high-fat diets (HFDs). HFDs increase the Firmicutes at the expense of the Bacteroidetes but KDs inhibit bifidobacterium growth short-term obesogenic HFD feeding but not KD causes an increase in fasting insulin and homeostatic model assessment-insulin resistance, reflecting the overall Actinobacteria phylum, Lactobacillus, which was significantly decreased. Earlier in this chapter, you learn that bifidobacterium and lactobacillus are a genus of gram-positive and you can see them in probiotic supplements as well. [272]

I search for more studies and research since the Keto diet is a hot topic nowadays. Many of you might see people do a keto diet and have a good result with weight loss in a short time period. I'm not anti keto and neither anti-fat. I love cheese, eggs, nuts, seeds, and avocado. However, I want to find out the facts and for long-term health benefits. If you are going to do a detox, the food you take in is supposed to be good for your internal organs and systems. I don't want to guide you for a quick fix and after that, go to fix something else along the line.

Study in 2018 comparison between High-fat diet and Keto diet effect on insulin sensitivity and blood glucose. The result.

1. Short-term HFD feeding, but not KD, causes an increase in fasting insulin and homeostatic model assessment-insulin resistance.

2. Short-term KD or HFD feeding causes impaired glucose clearance and insulin tolerance. KD induces more severe insulin resistance than a high-fat diet. [273]

All right, so now you know the answer. <u>The keto diet is not the one that is right for overall health.</u>

Feel free to read my endnote! As I said, I'm not anti-keto. If I can eat bacon and don't have any health problems I would love to eat as much as possible—however, the research has shown that it's harmful. In my 21 days sugar detox, you will have good fat, not low fat and not low carbs or high carb. It's a food combination that won't raise your blood sugar, benefit your gut and you don't store fat.

A study in 2021 for 16 weeks in mice showed a high-fat diet abundant in Omega-6 fatty acid (N-6 PUFA) changes the makeup of our gut microbiome—the collection of bacteria and viruses that live within our guts—resulting in an increased risk of intestinal disorders, sustains the gut growth of proinflammatory Mucispirillum schaedleri and Lactobacillus murinus. [274] Omega6 fatty acids is a polyunsaturated fatty acid from vegetable oils rich in linoleic acid, such as canola oil, corn oil, sunflower oil, safflower oil, and soybean oils.

High-fat diets have been affected by reduced gut microbiota richness, increased Firmicutes to Bacteroidetes ratio, and several changes in the family, genus, and species levels. Saturated (SFA), monounsaturated (MUFA), polyunsaturated (PUFA), and conjugated linoleic fatty acids share critical pathways of immune system activation/inhibition with gut microbes leading to obesity and inflammation. [275] [276] However, fat is not an enemy. You should consume fat with your calorie intake. Fat isn't created equal, just like carbohydrates and protein. A diet enriched in MUFA and PUFA increases the Bacteroidetes: Firmicutes ratio and elevates numbers of lactic acid bacteria—Bifidobacteria and Akkermansia muciniphila. Conversely, SFA (long-chain saturated fatty acids) promotes the growth of Bilophila and Faecalibacterium prausnitzii and causes a decline in Bifidobacterium, Bacteroidetes, Bacteroides, Prevotella, Lactobacillus spp.

WHY IS OMEGA-3 GOOD FOR YOUR GUT MICROBIOME?

Studies show Omega-3 affects the gut microbiome in three main ways:

1. Omega-3 increases in the Bacteroidetes, Lactobacillus, and butyrate-producing bacteria, and an abundance of gut microbes included lactic acids. [277]

2. Omega-3 alters the levels of proinflammatory mediators, such as endotoxins (lipopolysaccharides) and IL17. It's an excellent source of anti-inflammatory properties. It exerts a beneficial effect on various inflammation-related diseases, such as inflammatory bowel disease, rheumatoid arthritis, asthma, cancer, and cardiovascular diseases.

3. Omega-3 regulates the levels of short-chain fatty acids (SCFAs) or short-chain fatty acid salts. [278]

The addition of omega-3 to the diet could decrease LDL cholesterol, prevent myocardial infarction, and reduce the morbidity and mortality of cardiovascular disease. [279]

Omega-3 polyunsaturated fatty acids (PUFAs) include α-linolenic acid (ALA), stearidonic acid (SDA), eicosapentaenoic acid (EPA), docosapentaenoic acid (DPA), and docosahexaenoic acid (DHA). Oils containing these fatty acids (FAs), or some of these fatty acids, originate from certain plant sources or are changed in plants, as well as marine, algal, and single-cell sources. Long-chain (LC) omega-3 FAs such as EPA and DHA occur in the body lipids of fatty fish, the liver of lean white fish, and the blubber of marine mammals.

WHAT FOOD IS THE BEST SOURCE OF OMEGA-3?

Omega-3 FAs are only found in aquatic organisms and originate in the liver of lean white fish such as cod and halibut, the body of oily fish such as mackerel, menhaden, and salmon, and the specialized subcutaneous layer of fat of marine mammals such as seals and whales. The major Omega-3 from marine sources are EPA and DHA, and DPA is present in low levels in most fish oils. Marine oils are also rich sources of fat-soluble vitamins. The livers of cod, haddock, halibut, shark, whales, and tuna are used to produce vitamins A and D supplement oils. Vitamins A and D contents of cod liver oil are 1,000 and 10 IU/g. Among all fish oils, cod flesh, halibut, and skipjack tuna have been shown to contain the highest amounts of DHA (30% of total FAs), whereas cod flesh, flounder species, and haddock contain the highest amounts of EPA (15–19% of total FAs).

Check <u>Table 1 for more detail of EPA, DHA and DPA percentage.</u> Besides fish and marine mammals, crabs, lobster, shrimps, krill, prawns, crayfish, oysters, clams, mussels, scallops, squid, octopus, and cuttlefish also contain Omega-3.

Table 1. The omega-3 polyunsaturated fatty acid content of marine sources.

Marine sources	EPA(%)	DHA (%)	DPA(%)
Butterfish oil	5.1	10.8	2.4
Cod flesh oil	19.1	32.6	2
Cod liver oil	12.2	12.7	1.7
Haddock oil	14.8	24.8	1.9
Halibut oil	9.6	30.6	2.6
Herringing oil	7.5	6.8	0.75
Mackerel oil	8	19.3	1.6
Menhaden oil	18.3	9.6	1.8
Salmon oil	6.2	9.1	1.8
Skipjack tuna oil	11.1	29.1	0
Winter flounder oil	14.4	20.1	0
Yellowtail flounder oil	15	18.7	3.3
Seafood			
Blue mussel	19.6	13.2	0

Greenland cockle	22.6	16.5	0.1
Icelandic scallop	26.9	25.9	0
Lobster	17.04	7.69	1.29
Octopus	16.1	20.6	1.8
Red crab	12.13	11.93	2.25
Rock crab	20.74	10.35	2.06
Shrimp	15.26	11.37	0.74
Squid (European)	14.3	31.6	0.4
Squid	13.9	16.9	1.3
Surf clam	22.9	14.3	Trace

The primary source of ALA is plants, concentrated in some seeds and nuts and in some vegetable oils. Flaxseed, chia seeds, walnut, and echium seed oils are excellent sources of ALA, whereas safflower, sunflower, corn, and soybean oils are rich in linoleic acid. Flaxseed oil contains a high amount of ALA (49.2 g/100 g) than other sources. EPA and DHA can be synthesized in the human body using ALA as a precursor. However, in the human body, bioconversion of ALA to EPA and DHA is limited. The metabolic pathway of synthesis of Omega-3 from dietary ALA. SDA is the first metabolite synthesized from ALA, which leads to the synthesis of EPA, DPA, and DHA.

The Boraginaceae family, such as borage, Echium vulgare, Buglossoides arvensis (corn gromwell), hemp oil, and fish, are excellent sources of SDA. However, SDA is not a major component of the human diet.

Micro-algae and some microorganisms (fungi) also contain Omega-3. Marine algae are the predominant producers of Omega-3 worldwide in all ecosystems. Various algal species have been identified as sources of DHA. Crypthecodinium cohnii and Schizochytrium spp. are the two major algal sources of DHA at levels of 55% and 40% of total fatty acids. Omega-3, especially EPA and DHA, are synthesized by phytoplankton, and algae are transferred via the food web and deposited into the blood of fish and marine mammals. For this reason, fish, marine mammals, and seafood contain EPA and DHA. [280] [281]

If you don't eat fish and seafood, you can get ALA from plant sources, but you need to get EPA and DHA too. Therefore, algae oil is the best source of omega-3 for vegans and vegetarians. However, if you are going to buy an omega-3 supplement, now you know salmon oil is not the best source. *The number one Omega-3 supplement is algae oil because not only you get enough EPA and DHA, but you also avoid mercury, and it's the best choice for the world environment since now global fish stock is low.*

Sweet surprise

DHA from Omega-3 has prebiotic effects. A recent review showed that Omega-3 PUFA indirectly or directly modulates the gut microbiota, which reduces pro-inflammatory levels and increase short-chain fatty acids. [282] [283]

The best way to get Omega-3 is from food sources. If you can't get enough omega-3 from a food source, you can also get it from supplements.

> *My first choice is algae oil, the second is cod liver oil, the third, krill oil, and the fourth, fish oil and lastly salmon oil. Krill oil might have less EPA and DHA compared to fish and salmon oil, but the bioavailability of EPA + DHA from krill oil was higher than that of EPA + DHA from fish oil and salmon oil.*

The recommendation for Omega-3 in the United States is 70 mg/day (DHA and EPA) for 1-3 years old, 500 mg/day (DHA and EPA) for general adults, and 200 mg/day for pregnant and breastfeeding. Different countries have made recommendations for the Omega-3 intake differently. The RDI for DHA is between 70 to 250 mg/day or 40 to 2,300 mg/day in combination with other types of omega-3. The FDA has ruled that intakes of up to 3 g/d of marine omega-3 fatty acids are GRAS (Generally Recognized As Safe) to include in the diet. [284] [285] However, 450 mg of DHA showed greater cardiovascular risk reduction than any other supplement.[286]

If you eat salmon, mackerel, herring, and trout. These fish can provide about 0.68–1.43 g DHA per 100 g meat. Check the major dietary sources of EPA, DPA, and DHA are summarized in Table 2.

Table 2 Food source of Omega-3 per 100-gram meat. [287]

Food	EPA	DPA	DHA	Combined DPA +DHA
Anchovy	763	41	1292	2055
Beef	2	4	1	3
Blue crab	101	9	67	168
Bluefish	323	79	665	988
Catfish, farmed	20	18	69	89
Clams	138	104	146	284
Chicken breast	10	10	20	30
Cod, Pacific	42	5	118	160
Eggs	0	7	58	58
Flounder and sole	168	34	132	300
Grouper	35	17	213	248
Halibut	80	20	155	235
Herring, Atlantic	909	71	1105	2014
King mackerel	174	22	227	401
Lobster	117	6	78	195

Mackerel, Atlantic	504	106	699	1203
Mussels	276	44	506	782
Oysters, wild	274	16	210	484
Pollock, Atlantic	91	28	451	542
Pork	0	10	2	2
Salmon, farmed	862	393	1104	1966
Salmon, wild	411	368	1429	1840
Sardines, Atlantic	473	0	509	982
Scallops	72	5	104	176
Shrimp	50	5	52	102
Snapper	48	22	273	321
Striped bass	169	0	585	754
Swordfish	127	168	772	899
Trout	259	235	677	936
Tuna, light (skipjack)	91	17	237	328
Tuna, white (albacore)	233	18	629	862

A study in 2017 reveals that "The consumption of two healthy diets (Mediterranean (MED) with 35% of calories as fat (22% MUFA fat,

6% PUFA fat and <10% saturated fat) or low-fat diet (LF) with <30% total fat (<10% saturated fat, 12%–14% MUFA fat and 6–8% PUFA fat) may restore the gut microbiome dysbiosis in obese patients with coronary heart disease. [288]

In conclusion, a High-Fat Diet Induces Gut Microbiome Dysbiosis and Colonic Inflammation. However, we need fat for our body function, but keep in mind that all oils are processed, so it's better to consume fat from seeds, nuts, and fruits, i.e., avocado and durian, and use extra virgin olive oil and coconut oil sparingly when you need oil for cooking. Consuming omega-3 more than omega 6 and omega 9 from food sources would be beneficial for your gut microbiome and your overall health. The ratio of omega 3: 6:9 should be 3:2:1.

6. Pesticides, Glyphosate herbicide, and GMOs

Pesticides are chemical substances that kill pests. A pesticide is a chemical or a biological agent such as a virus, bacterium, antimicrobial, or disinfectant that deters, incapacitates, kills, and pests.

Types of Pesticides

These are grouped according to the pests which they kill:

Insecticides–insects

Herbicides–plants

Rodenticides–rodents (rats & mice)

Bactericides–bacteria

Fungicides–fungi

Larvicides–larvae [289]

HOW PESTICIDES, GLYPHOSATE HERBICIDES, AND GMOS AFFECT THE GUT

Roundup is a weed killer, and it's a very popular herbicide produced by biotech giant Monsanto and was first established in 1974. The key element in Roundup is glyphosate. Glyphosate is also used in many other herbicides. Glyphosate-based herbicides (GBIIs) are the most frequently used herbicides in agriculture, forestry management, cities, and private homeowners. In 2015, the World Health Organization (WHO) declared glyphosate has the potential to cause cancer.

The study in 2020 in Japanese quail females and males reported that GBH exposure altered overall gut microbiome composition, especially at a younger age and in females, and suppressed potentially beneficial microbes at an early age. It decreased male testosterone in all ages but did not influence reproduction. [290]

Another study in 2019 reviewed the impact of Glyphosate induced intestinal dysbiosis on the central nervous system, focusing on emotional, neurological, and neurodegenerative disorders. A wide variety of factors was investigated in relation to brain-related changes. [291]

The study in 2020, "The Effect of Pesticides on the Microbiome of Animals," showed that pesticides could affect various parameters of the animal microbiome, such as the taxonomic composition of bacteria, bacterial biodiversity, and bacterial ratios, and change the microbiome of multiple organisms from insects to mammals. Pesticide induced changes in the microbiome, reducing the animal's immunity, reproductive ability, and even their behavioral characteristics. Pesticides have a significant effect on the taxonomic composition and ratio of bacteria in the gut of bumblebees and bees.[292]

If you live on a farm or close to a farm that uses pesticides, you have a better chance of getting the harmful substance. However, all of risk of getting this chemical from food. The major foods that contain glyphosate are genetically modified (GM), glyphosate-resistant crops, such as corn, canola, soybeans, alfalfa and sugar beets.[293]

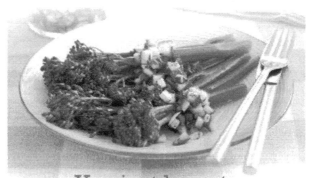

You don't have to
EAT LESS

You just have to
EAT RIGHT

HOW CAN YOU AVOID THIS HARMFUL CHEMICAL?

1. **Consuming non-GMO products**. You can check out the label of the non-GMO project verified. For more information, you can check out the website. https://www.nongmoproject.org/

2. **Check out the dirty dozen list and clean fifteen** from the Environment working group (EWG). You can buy non organic produce from the clean fifteen list and buy the organic produce from the dirty dozen list.

The 2021 Dirty Dozen List

1. Strawberries

2. Spinach

3. Kale, collard greens, and mustard greens

4. Nectarines

5. Apples

6. Grapes

7. Cherries

8. Peaches

9. Pears

10. Bell and hot peppers

11. Celery

12. Tomatoes

The 2021 Clean Fifteen

1. Avocados

2. Sweet corn

3. Pineapple

4. Onions

5. Papaya

6. Sweet peas (frozen)

7. Eggplant

8. Asparagus

9. Broccoli

10. Cabbage

11. Kiwi

12. Cauliflower

13. Mushrooms

14. Honeydew melon

15. Cantaloupe

3. Consuming organic food

Yes, organic is the best. Do you know what is different between an organic product and non-GMO?

Organic food

- Grown or farmed without the use of artificial chemicals, hormones, antibiotics, genetically modified organisms (GMOs), and pesticides.

- Organically grown crops have more specific vitamins, minerals, and antioxidants and less nitrate, which are associated with an increased risk of certain types of cancer.

- Animals raised organically aren't treated with growth hormones, antibiotics, or artificial drugs.

- Free of artificial food additives. This includes artificial sweeteners, preservatives, coloring, flavoring, and monosodium glutamate (MSG).

Non-GMO food

- GMO stands for "genetically modified organism."

- Non-GMO means that the genetic makeup of the plants and animals used in the product has not been altered for food production.

- But Non-GMO is not organic; non-GMO foods may still be produced using pesticides, hormones, antibiotics, and artificial preservatives and colorings. However, organic food is non-GMO.

HOW TO CHECK OUT PLU CODES

If you can't buy organic fruits and vegetables, you can check out the PLU codes. PLU or Price Look-Up codes have been used by supermarkets since 1990 to make check-out and inventory control easier, faster, and more accurate. [294]

- The 4-digit codes, starting with 3 or 4, are for conventionally grown produce. For example, 3590 or 4901.

- The 5-digit codes, starting with 9, are used to identify organic produce. For example, 97610.

- The 5-digit codes, starting with 8, are genetically modified. 86451

In conclusion, it's a good idea to avoid GMO crops because it's not worth your health with pesticides, and it's even better if you can choose organic products.

> *Sweet surprise*
>
> *Exercise determines an increase in good bacteria, such as bacteria producing lactic acid (e.g., Bifidobacteria and Lactobacillus), which modulates mucosal immunity and prevents pathogens invasion, or Blautia coccoides and Eubacterium rectale, which convert lactate into butyrate.[295]*

ACTIVITIES THAT KILL YOUR GUT MICROBIOME

1. Loss of sleep

Many evidence shows that circadian rhythm disorders, insomnia, and loss of sleep are linked to a range of health problems, including obesity, diabetes, metabolic syndrome, and inflammatory diseases. Over 50% of patients with IBS have comorbid depression, anxiety, or sleep problems. Loss of sleep affects the balance of the gut microbiome. However, this is like a chicken and egg situation. Gut microbiome imbalance also causes problems with sleeping and moods.

Both interrupted sleep and short sleep duration are associated with gut dysbiosis, which may be because of activation of the HPA-axis.

[296] HPA stands for the hypothalamic-pituitary-adrenal, and HPA-axis is central to homeostasis, stress responses, energy metabolism, and neuropsychiatric function. [297]

Many studies have identified a microbiome-gut-brain (MGB) axis. Within this axis, the microbiota in the gut affects brain function through 3 pathways that produce a bidirectional flow of information.

1. The immunoregulatory pathway, in which the microbiota interact with immune cells in such a way as to affect the levels of cytokines, cytokinetic reaction factor, and prostaglandin E2. As a result, brain function is affected.

2. The neuroendocrine pathway. There are over 20 types of enteroendocrine cells in the intestine, which make up the largest endocrine organ in the human body. The gut microbiome may affect the hypothalamic-pituitary-adrenal (HPA) axis and the central nervous system (CNS) by regulating the secretion of neurotransmitters, such as cortisol, tryptophan, and serotonin (5-HT).

3. The vagus nerve pathway, in which the enteric nervous system plays an important role.

Microbial metabolism produces a variety of neurotransmitters, cytokines, and metabolites such as serotonin (5-HT), dopamine (DA), GABA, short-chain fatty acids (SCFAs), melatonin, and other compounds.

90% of the serotonin (5-HT) in the human body is derived from chromaffin cells in the gastroenteric tract and some gut bacteria. About 50% of dopamine is produced in the gastrointestinal tract by enteric neurons and intestinal epithelial cells. Lactobacillus and Bifidobacterium can secrete GABA, and abnormal expression of GABA mRNA is often observed in patients with depression and insomnia.

In conclusion, there is a bidirectional connection between the gut microbiome and sleep. Inflammation and endocrine hormones play essential roles in this process. The chronic disturbances of host circadian rhythms, sleep loss, and depression have an impact on the metabolism of indigenous gut bacteria and trigger changes in their composition, reducing the total number of organisms of the Lactobacillaceae family but increasing the populations of Bacteroides multiforme, Enterococci, the Lachnospiraceae, and the Ruminococcaceae, which causes microbial dysbiosis. [298] [299] You should try to get better sleep by putting away the electronic device an hour before your bedtime and relaxing. Do not invite stress to your bedroom. Sometimes it's hard to do, but please try your best. Try to go to bed on time like you have an appointment and if you travel to a different time zone, adjust your mealtime and sleep time according to your destination a day in advance or during your flight.

2. Smoking

Cigarette smoke is a toxic chemical hazard to a person who smokes and people around the smoker. The adverse effects of cigarette smoking are interfered by its impact on both nerve cell and immune-inflammatory systems. Cigarette smoking also is a major risk factor for intestinal disorders, such as Crohn's disease and peptic ulcer. The effects of cigarette smoking on intestinal disorders include changes in intestinal irrigation and microbiome, increases in permeability of the mucosa, and impaired mucosal immune responses.

Study in 2021 published that cigarette smoking increases the phylum of Bacteroidetes and decreases the variety of Firmicutes and

Proteobacteria in current smokers compared with never smokers. In a rat model, cigarette smoking decreases the concentrations of several organic acids, such as acetic acid, propionic acid, butyric acid, and valeric acid, and the population of Bifidobacterium in the cecum. Exposure to cigarette smoke elevates the intestinal pH, which benefits some bacteria, enabling them to thrive and cause intestinal microbiota dysbiosis. Dysbiosis of the intestinal microbiota may contribute to the pathogenesis of IBD, and patients with IBD have greater adherent bacteria numbers than healthy persons.[300]

3. Stress

The gut-brain axis (GBA) is relevant not only to these transient states but also to longer-lasting conditions. The gut-brain axis (GBA) is a bidirectional relationship between the central nervous system (CNS) and the enteric nervous system (ENS) of the body. It involves direct and indirect pathways. Digestive disorders, such as irritable bowel syndrome, coincide with mood disorders. Both chronic and acute stressors can shift the gut bacteria in multiple regions and habitats — both the inside (lumen) and border (mucosal lining) of the gut. Rodent research shows that stress can rapidly affect the gut bacteria's composition.[301] [302]

Study in 2019 revealed "stress and depression can increase gut barrier permeability. The result, a 'leaky gut,' allows bacteria to seep into circulation, producing an inflammatory response. Indeed, both depression and stress can provoke heightened inflammation and gut leakiness. [303]

All links from sleep, stress, gut, mood, brain, and overall health. You may not know where to get started first. All parts might be broken. I want to tell you; We are going to get a start with food after reading this book. After that, your mood, sleep, brain, and overall health will follow.

In Conclusion

Now you know what benefits the gut microbiome and what does not. In terms of macronutrient profiles, which predict unique gut microbiota populations, honestly, plant protein, unsaturated fats, and fiber support a pro-health gut microbiota — in contrast to excessive consumption of animal protein, saturated fats, and simple or artificial sugars. The Western diet, high in saturated fat, processed foods, and refined sugar, low gut microbiota diversity, and greater gut leakiness, which may contribute to metabolic syndrome and chronic disease onset.

In this sugar detox plan, you will devote your food in flavor to the gut microbiome. Remember to feed them good food. You will get a wonderful benefit from them, just like karma. In the next chapter, you will learn about the polyphenol foods that the gut microbiome loves so much. Polyphenols-rich food is not for wine, grapes, and berries, but more.

TO-DO LIST

Before you are going to read chapter 7.

1. Have a glass of your favorite red wine.

2. Have a small piece of chocolate.

3. Have a serving of your favorite fruit if you don't drink wine.

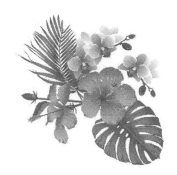

CHAPTER 7

POLYPHENOL-RICH FOODS MATTER TO YOUR WAISTLINE AND BRAIN CHEMISTRY

All plants have fiber. Some types of fiber are prebiotics, which are food for bacteria in the intestine. Once we feed the fiber to the bacteria in the colon, they are happy because they got the food. Then they multiply, and these are anti-inflammatory microbes. We feed them the right food. They will be happy and thank us by producing SCFAs. Every day, your gut microbiome needs food to survive and thrive. So, if you focus on a high fat or high protein diet, they will die off. Apart from fiber that your gut microbiome loves, polyphenol-rich food would be the best food for them.

WHY ARE POLYPHENOL-RICH FOODS GOOD FOR YOUR GUT?

Nature created the vibrant color of vegetables, fruits, and plants on purpose. The excellent, bright colors and unique flavors of fruits and vegetables are associated with phytochemicals. They contain essential vitamins and minerals that are micronutrients our body requires for functioning.

Clinical studies suggest polyphenols have prebiotic properties and antimicrobial activities against pathogenic gut microflora. [304]

Polyphenols have low absorption in the small intestine (less than 10%). Therefore, the unabsorbed polyphenols accumulate in the large intestine, and the gut microbiome turns these polyphenols into bioavailable products.

Research has shown that polyphenols can change the ecology of the gut microbiota (GM) by employing antimicrobial activity or prebiotic-like action against harmful gut bacteria living in the gut. Polyphenols expand the population of profitable species such as *Bifidobacterium and Lactobacillus,* which protect the intestinal barrier. They can increase the content of *Faecalibacterium prausnitzii,* characterized by an anti-inflammatory effect, and *Roseburia sp.,* which produces butyrate. Research confirms the influence of polyphenols on the content of *Akkermansia muciniphila* in the gut microbiota (GM). They exhibit a beneficial anti-inflammatory effect and a positive effect in preventing obesity. [305]

THE HEALTH BENEFIT OF POLYPHENOL-RICH FOODS

Polyphenols are a large group of occurring plant crops that provide various health benefits, such as.

1. Lower fasting blood sugar levels and increased insulin sensitivity are important components in cutting down your risk of type 2 diabetes. Among polyphenols, studies show anthocyanins may provide the most impressive antidiabetic effect. [306] [307] They're found in blue, purple, and red fruits, roots, flowers, and plants, such as a variety of berries, purple grapes, red hibiscus, red roses, and blackcurrants. [308]

2. Polyphenols have powerful antioxidant and anti-inflammatory effects, [309] [310] both of which can be beneficial for cancer

prevention. [311] From studies, polyphenols, especially in combination with other polyphenols or micronutrients, have been effective against multiple targets in cancer development and progression and should be safe and effective approaches to cancer prevention and therapy. [312]

3. The antioxidant properties of polyphenols help reduce chronic inflammation, a risk factor for heart disease and help lower blood pressure and lower LDL (bad) cholesterol levels, as well as higher HDL (good) cholesterol. [313] [314]

4. Polyphenols improve digestion by promoting the growth of good gut bacteria while fending off bad ones. [315]

> ### Sweet surprise
>
> *From the research, polyphenol-rich tea extracts can promote the production of beneficial bifidobacteria, besides green tea polyphenols may help combat harmful bacteria, such as E. Coli, C. difficile, and Salmonella, and also improve symptoms of inflammatory bowel disease (IBD). [316]*

5. Polyphenol-rich foods may boost your focus and memory. The research found that cacao may enhance blood flow to the brain and has identified these polyphenols to increase working memory and attention. [317] [318] The impressive polyphenol ellagic acid (EA) not only has the properties of antioxidant, anti-inflammatory, anticancer, anti-diabetic, and cardio protection activities. EA is linked with the protection of neuronal abnormalities like anti-depressants, anti-anxiety, anti-nociception. Because Ellagic acid inhibits β-secretase enzymatic activities, it prevents the main pathologic hallmark of Alzheimer's disease (AD) as well. [319]

6. Polyphenol helps to protect you from ultraviolet radiation. [320]
Ultraviolet (UV) radiation is a known cause of skin cancer, skin aging, eye damage and may affect the immune system.

POLYPHENOL-RICH FOODS ARE NOT ONLY GRAPES, BERRIES, AND WINE

Polyphenols are present in foods and beverages of plant origins (e.g., fruits, vegetables, spices, soy, legumes, nuts, tea, and wine).

Based on chemical structures, natural polyphenols can be divided into five classes, including flavonoids, phenolic acids, lignans, stilbenes, and other polyphenols.

Flavonoids and phenolic acids are the most common classes and account for about 60% and 30% of all natural polyphenols. [321] Look at table 1 for more detail.

TABLE 1 THE CLASSIFICATION OF NATURAL POLYPHENOLS.

Classification		Representative Members	Major Dietary Sources
flavonoids	anthocyanins	delphinidin, pelargonidin, cyanidin, malvidin	berries, grapes, cherries, plums, pomegranates
	flavanols	epicatechin, epigallocatechin, EGCG, procyanidins	apples, pears, legumes, tea, cocoa, wine
	flavanones	hesperidin, naringenin	citrus fruits

	flavones	apigenin, chrysin, luteolin,	parsley, celery, orange, onions, tea, honey, spices
	flavonols	quercetin, kaempferol, myricetin, isorhamnetin, galangin	berries, apples, broccoli, beans, tea
	isoflavonoids	genistein, daidzein	soy
phenolic acids	hydroxybenzoic acid	ellagic acid, gallic acid	pomegranate, grapes, berries, walnuts, chocolate, wine, green tea
	hydroxycinnamic acid	ferulic acid, chlorogenic acid	coffee, cereal grains
lignans		sesamin, secoisolariciresinol diglucoside	flaxseeds, sesame
stilbenes		resveratrol, pterostilbene, piceatannol	grapes, berries, red wine

Have you ever wondered how people who live in tropical climates find food with polyphenol? They don't have berries, and they might not be able to afford red wine. Do they have access to polyphenol-rich food? The answer is yes. We often hear that polyphenol-rich food is red wine, grapes, and berries. But many foods have polyphenol.

Major polyphenol pigments in plants are anthocyanins, which exhibit red, purple, or blue color, and, to a lesser extent, the yellow flavonols and flavones. [322]

Flavones have a yellowish or cream color and also absorb ultraviolet light, so they can provide protection against UV radiation. People who live in the tropics can have access to yellow fruits, and they help with UV protection. You see how smart nature is.

I'm sharing my knowledge with you about polyphenol. You might see no one write this information, but it's fascinating to find out this information for me. Polyphenols are one reason that supports an excellent idea of eating natural rainbow fruits and vegetables. You know it's not only green that is good for you, but it's also a bright color or its white color. Nature creates them for your health and vitality. So now, when you have food or even a smoothie, you should think about the colorful food that protects and prevents you from disease and also helps you lose weight and boost immunity.

From table 1, based on chemical structures, natural polyphenols can be divided into five classes, including flavonoids, phenolic acids, lignans, stilbenes, and other polyphenols.

1. **Flavonoids.**

The term is derived from the Latin word "flavus," meaning yellow. They have subgroups: anthocyanins, flavonols, flavanones, flavones, flavanols or catechins, and isoflavonoid.

1.1 Anthocyanins are the basis of the bright, attractive red, blue and purple colors of fruits and vegetables. You can find them from berries such as strawberries, blueberries, blackberries, blackcurrant, redcurrant, and raspberries, with levels ranging from about 100 to about 700 mg/100 g of the fresh product, but the highest content is found in elderberries and chokeberries, which can contain up to 1.4-1.8 g of anthocyanins per 100 g of product. Other good sources of anthocyanins include purple corn, cherries, plums, cranberry, pomegranate, eggplant, black rice, wine, grapes, purple sweet potatoes, black beans, prunes, roselle, and red/purple vegetables such as black carrots, red cabbage, radish, and purple cauliflower. [323]

1.2 Flavonols, the subgroup flavonols are kaempferol, quercetin, myricetin, isorhamnetin and galangin.

First one that I want to give a spotlight to is **kaempferol.** Many studies have described the beneficial effects of dietary kaempferol in reducing the risk of chronic diseases, especially cancer.[324]

The top 10 most kaempferol-dense vegetables.

1. Watercress
2. Mustard green
3. Arugula
4. New Zealand spinach
5. Kale
6. Endive
7. Radish seeds
8. Dock
9. Garden cress
10. Turnip greens

The top 10 most kaempferol-dense fruits.[325]

1. Blueberry
2. Gooseberry
3. Watermelon

4. Kiwi

5. Strawberry

6. Apricot

7. Elderberry

8. Blackberry

9. Peach

10. Cherry

Kaempferol is found in plants or botanical products used in traditional medicine such as ginkgo biloba, lime horsetail, Moringa, the Japanese pagoda tree, and propolis (a compound produced by bees).

Sweet surprise

Curcumin is a flavonoid from the rhizome of Turmeric (Curcuma longa) belongs to the family Zingiberaceae which is native to Southeast Asia countries. You can see it in Southeast Asia and Middle Eastern dishes. Curcumin has good therapeutic and preventive potential against several major human conditions, such as cardiovascular, inflammation suppression, antimicrobial, obesity, tumorigenesis, chronic tiredness, antidepressant & neurological function, anxiety, muscle & bone loss, and neuropathic pain. Phytochemical composition of turmeric polyphenol includes 0.4% saponin, 0.76% alkaloid, 0.03% sterol, 1.08% tannin, 0.40% flavonoid, 0.82% phytic acid, and 0.08% phenol. 326 Turmeric is one of the magical herbs on the planet that you shouldn't miss.

Quercetin comes from the Latin word "Quercetum", which means Oak Forest. It is one of the most widely used bioflavonoids in the treatment of metabolic and inflammatory disorders. Quercetin cannot be produced in the human body. It has an interesting profile of antioxidant properties, has been used as a nutritional supplement, and may be beneficial to a variety of diseases. Some of the beneficial effects include cardiovascular protection, anticancer, antitumor, anti-ulcer, anti-allergy, anti-viral, anti-inflammatory activity, anti-diabetic, gastroprotective effects, anti-hypertension, immunomodulatory and anti-infective. [327] Recently, many studies have found quercetin has great potential for treatment Covid-19 or SARS-CoV-2. [328] [329] [330]

Quercetin is present in different food sources such as mango, plums, cranberry, blueberry, chokeberry, buckwheat, honey, beans, lettuce, chicory, onion in different amounts of chemical structure.

TABLE 2 THE TOP 20 MOST QUERCETIN-DENSE FOODS

Food source (100 g.) [331]	Quercetin content(mg.)
1. Canned caper	180.76
2. Raw lovage leave	170.01
3. Raw dock leave	86.24
4. Fresh dill	55.13
5. Hot wax raw yellow pepper or Hungarian wax pepper	50.62
6. Ancho pepper	27.61
7. Corn poppy leave	26.31
8. Buckwheat	23.08
9. Raw cowberry (lingonberry)	21.01
10. Sweet potato raw leave	20.55
11. Dry unsweetened cocoa powder	20.14
12. Red raw onion	19.94
13. Boiled onions	19.37
14. Wild frozen whortleberries	17.71

15. Hot green raw chili pepper	16.81
16. Raw cranberry juice	16.42
17. Serrano raw pepper	15.96
18. Spring raw onion	14.23
19. Raw cranberry	14.01
20. Lingo raw berry	12.17

It's so many foods that have quercetin, but they are in a small amount. For example, the popular kale has 7.72 mg of quercetin /100 g. You probably eat 100 grams of kale rather than 100 grams of dill, right? Remember, variety is the key to feeding different gut microbiomes.

Sweet surprise

Onion is another impressive vegetable in the allium family, and it is one of the oldest cultivated plants used worldwide as both vegetable and flavoring. Onion contains sulfur amino acids together with many vitamins and minerals, one of that is B vitamins, including Thiamin (B1), Riboflavin (B2), Niacin (B3), Pantothenic acid (B5), pyridoxine (B6), folate (B9) — which play key roles in metabolism, red blood cell production and nerve function. It's also high in vitamin C, the powerful antioxidant and rich source of potassium. Onions contain flavonoid antioxidants, quercetin compounds that decrease triglycerides and anti-inflammation, low cholesterol levels — all of which may reduce heart disease risk and lower blood pressure. It helps control blood sugar, which is especially significant for people with diabetes or prediabetes. 332 333

Studies show a sulfur-containing compound in onions that has been shown to decrease tumor development and slow the spread of ovarian and lung cancer.334 The antibacterial properties in onions can support you to fight dangerous bacteria, such as Escherichia coli (E. coli), Pseudomonas aeruginosa, Staphylococcus aureus (S. aureus) and

Bacillus cereus. [335] [336] Onions can promote your digestive system as well since they are a rich source of fiber and prebiotics, which are beneficial for gut microbes and its fundamental for optimal gut health. Onions are especially rich in prebiotic inulin and fructooligosaccharides. [337] This helps develop the number of friendly bacteria in your gut and enhance immune function.

Myricetin can help you lose weight, reduce visceral fat and cholesterol

You might not have heard of it before. Most people know resveratrol from red wine is good, but polyphenols have so many chemical compounds that have significant benefits for your health. This is one of them that most people don't know. Highlight myricetin could reduce weight gain, visceral fat, and cholesterol. It also has anti-diabetes properties. [338] [339] The science publication in 2020 revealed that myricetin has antimicrobial, antioxidant, neuroprotective, antidiabetic, anticancer, immunomodulatory, cardioprotective, analgesic, anti-hypertensive properties and also wound healing potential.[340] You can check out the myricetin rich food from the table below.

TABLE 3 MYRICETIN (MG/100 G) RICH FOODS

1.	Cranberry	6600
2.	Dock	5700
3.	Sweet potato leaves	4400
4.	Chard, swiss	3100
5.	Broad Beans, immature seeds	2600

6. Rutabagas	2100
7. Garlic	1600
8. Blueberry	1300
9. Peppers, hot chili, green	1200
10. Blackberry	700
11. Lotus root	600
12. Lemon	500

Source: USDA Food Database (compiled data from all fruits and vegetables that contain information on myricetin concentration)

Sweet surprise

Garlic is an excellent medicinal plant owing to its preventive aspects in cardiovascular diseases, regulating blood pressure, lowering blood sugar and cholesterol levels. It's antibacterial, antiviral, antifungal and antiparasitic, enhancing the immune system and having antitumoral, and antioxidant qualities. Garlic contains sulfur compounds (allicin, alliin and, agony). Allicin is an organic compound that has antimicrobial, antiviral and antibacterial properties. 341 Garlic is considered a functional spice because of its diverse array of nutritional constituents, phytochemicals, and fiber. It contains high levels of potassium, phosphorus, zinc, and sulfur, moderate levels of selenium, calcium, magnesium, manganese, iron, and low levels of sodium, vitamin A and C and B-complex. Its main bioactive compounds, particularly polyphenols, flavonoids, flavanols, tannins, saponins, polysaccharides, sulfur-containing compounds (including alliin, allicin), enzymes (like alliinase, peroxidase, myrosinase), and other compounds, such as β-phellandrene, phellandrene, citral, linalool, and geraniol.

There are over twenty well-known polyphenolic compounds in garlic, including kaempferol 3,7-di-O-rhamnoside, kaempferol-3 glucuronide, kaempferol-3-O-glucoside, kaempferol-3-O-beta-d-glucoside-7-O-alpha-l-rhamnoside, luteolin, and apigenin. It contains 17 amino acids with eight main amino acids. 342 So eating garlic every day keeps the doctor away!

Next is **galangin**. Most people might not have heard of galangal, but I'm familiar with it. I grew up in a Thai household, and we use galangal in many Thai dishes such as red curry, jungle curry, choo chii, tom yam, and tom kha.

Galangal root is rich in polyphenols, a group of antioxidants and antimicrobial [343] [344] linked to health benefits such as lower blood sugar and LDL (bad) cholesterol levels, protect your cells from damaging free radicals, improved memory, protect against type 2 diabetes, heart disease and mental decline. [345] [346] [347] [348] Many studies suggest the active compound in galangal root has anti-cancer effects on several cancers, including skin cancer, liver cancer, colon cancer cell, breast cancer, stomach cancer, pancreatic cancer, and leukemia cells. [349] [350] [351] [352] [353] [354] [355] [356] Thanks to the phytochemical of galangal compounds including tannins, alkaloids, flavonoids, and saponins, it showed significant antibacterial, and antimicrobial activity. Galangal roots kill harmful bacteria, such as the B. cereus, Staph. aureas, P. aeruginosa and E. coli. [357] [358] You should try galangal if you have lower back pain or knee injury. Many researchers discovered galangal reduces disease-causing inflammation, as it contains HMP, an occurring phytochemical. So, it can reduce chronic pain and inflammation. One study also showed that a purified ginger and galangal extract had a significant effect on reducing symptoms in patients with osteoarthritis (OA) of the knee. [359] [360] [361] [362] [363]

Sweet surprise

Ginger is the ingredient that I always saw in the kitchen where I grew up in Thailand. The main polyphenol constituents identified in the ginger extract are 6-, 8-, and 10-gingerol and 6-shogaol in the digestive fluids. 364 Ginger solves many problems such as digestion, nausea, especially morning sickness, reducing menstrual discomfort, and it's an herbal remedy for colds. Ginger has all the cover for all kinds of health issues. The plant has several chemicals responsible for its medicinal properties, such as anti-arthritis, anti-inflammatory, antidiabetic, antibacterial, antifungal, and anticancer. 365 Of course, ginger can help you drop weight. A study in 2019 reviewed that ginger decreased bodyweight, the waist-hip ratio, the hip ratio, fasting glucose, and increased HDL - good cholesterol among people with overweight. 366Other studies discovered that the antioxidants and bioactive compounds in ginger could inhibit inflammatory responses that develop in the brain. Ginger can help enhance brain function and protect against Alzheimer's disease.367

1.3 Flavanols, the subgroups are epicatechin, epigallocatechin, EGCG, and procyanidins. Flavanols occur abundantly in tea leaves (green tea, 25–35% in dry leaves), cocoa beans, and grape seeds. In addition, they are found in many fruits like grapes, apples, apricots, and different berries.

Epigallocatechin gallate (EGCG) is a unique plant compound that gets a lot of attention for its positive impact on health. EGCG is predominantly found in green tea. It also exists in small amounts in other foods, such as in white tea, black teas, oolong tea, pecans, pistachios, hazelnuts, as well as in fruits such as cranberries, apples, cherries, strawberries, blackberries, kiwis, pears, peaches, and avocados. [368]

EGCG is the most abundant and powerful antioxidant in green tea, and extensive research has shown that it has significant antioxidant, anti-cancer, anti-microbial, and neuroprotective properties and has therapeutic potential against various human diseases. [369]

Now you see polyphenol is not only red wine, grapes and berries. It's all good stuff here. Now you understand more and more. Everything is making sense. Why is polyphenol good for the gut and all superfoods, and healthy food all contain polyphenols?

1.4 Flavanone appears at high concentrations in tomatoes and citrus and certain aromatic plants, such as mint.

The main compounds are *naringenin* in grapefruit, *hesperetin* in oranges, lemons, limes, tangerines, and other fruits, such as grapes and *eriodictyol* in lemons. [370]

Hesperidin is found in lemons, sweet oranges, lemons, limes, tangerines. Its well-known benefits for cardiovascular function, type II diabetes, and anti-inflammation. Recent studies have shown multiple benefits of hesperidin for cutaneous functions, including wound healing, UV protection, anti-inflammation, antimicrobial, anti- skin cancer, and skin lightening. [371]

Bergamot is one of the interesting fruits in clinical practice as a treatment for high cholesterol, anti-diabetic and moderate hyperglycemia in metabolic syndrome. The main compounds of bergamot are neo eriocitrin, neohesperidin, naringin, melitidin and brutieridin. [372] Bergamot also has antimicrobials, antioxidant, and anti-inflammatory properties. [373] [374] You might see it in essential oil or supplement form to speed up healing of mouth ulcers, cold sores, and herpes, help relieve symptoms with bacterial infections, fight against fungal infections and also help to reduce anxiety and stress.

After you read this part, now you can share your knowledge with your friends and family that polyphenol is not only grape, wine, and berries, but it has plenty of yellow and orange color like citrus fruits. In

Thailand, we can find so many types of oranges and enjoy different tastes and flavors. The genus Citrus belongs to the family Rutaceae, including about 140 genera and 1300 species. Citrus combines species like orange, lemon, grapefruit, bergamot, yuzu, and kumquat as diverse tropical fruit. I know they are a big family. Several studies showed the various beneficial activities of Citrus and its antioxidant, antimicrobial, anti-inflammatory, controlling insect properties.[375]

1.5 Flavones, in food, contain apigenin *and luteolin*. Important dietary sources of flavones are parsley and celery.

Apigenin is a common flavonoid distributed in plant-based food, such as orange, parsley, onions, tea, and wheat sprouts. Luteolin is abundant in artichoke and several spices, including sage, thyme, and oregano.

1.6 Isoflavonoids are plant-based secondary metabolites abundant in plant species that belong to Papilionoideae, a subfamily of Leguminosae. Examples of most studied isoflavones include biochanin A, genistein, daidzein, glycitein and formononetin. You don't need to remember all of this, but I just added the name for reference and just in case for further studies for some of you.

Soy and its products and legume seeds (lentils, beans, peas) are one of the richest sources of isoflavone. Soybean seeds are an essential source that contains a massive amount of isoflavonoids in the human diet. However, the primary sources of isoflavone are legumes, the Fabaceae family in soy, and red clover. Isoflavone can also be found in trace quantities in some fruits, such as strawberries and apples. Isoflavonoids are derived phytoestrogen compounds that have been reported for antidiabetic effects through multiple research studies. [376] The health benefits of isoflavonoids have increased because of a variety of bioprotective effects, including antioxidant, antimutagenic, anticancer, antiproliferative activities.

Isoflavonoids have been defined as dietary antioxidants, i.e., compounds that may protect against oxidative stress linked to inflammation and the risk of macromolecule damage by free radicals and by related oxygen and nitrogen-based oxidizing agents. They may protect the body from hormone-related cancers, like breast, uterus, and prostate. Also, a wide spectrum of health-protective abilities that have been attributed to them, e.g., immune response, risk reduction of chronic diseases including cardiovascular diseases, diabetes, cancer, osteoporosis, and obesity, as well as relief of menopausal symptoms. [377] So now you know eating soy, beans, lentils, and peas is super good for your health.

The next group of polyphenols is phenolic acid.

2. Phenolic acid

Two important types of phenolic acids are hydroxy benzoic acids and hydroxy cinnamic acids.

2.1 Hydroxy benzoic acid

Most people might not have heard of hydroxy benzoic acid, but once I mentioned ellagic acid and gallic acid. You might have heard of it.

Ellagic acid is one of the well- studied phytochemicals for powerful anti-inflammatory, cancer-fighting properties, and it may be useful for the treatment and prevention of conditions like cancer, type 2 diabetes, and Alzheimer's. [378] [379] [380] You can find Ellagic acid polyphenols in fruits and vegetables, including blackberries, raspberries, strawberries, cranberries, cloudberry, tree nuts (walnuts, pistachios, cashews, acorns, and pecans), pomegranates, persimmon, plum, peach, muscadine grapes, and goji berry. [381] New study in 2020 found Korean black raspberries with major bioactive compounds, ellagic acid, also decrease cholesterol levels.[382]

Gallic acid **(GA)** has many biological properties, including antioxidant, anticancer, anti-inflammatory, and antimicrobial properties. Recent studies have shown that GA and its derivatives not only enhance gut microbiome (GM) activities but also modulate immune responses. GA compound can be found in grapes, pomegranates, tea leaves, and gallnuts.[383]

What are gallnuts? It's very interesting to find that gallnuts are a group of very special natural products formed through parasitic interaction between plants and insects. It has been used in traditional Chinese medicine to cure cancer for centuries.[384]

2.2 Hydroxy cinnamic acid

Several simple phenolic compounds, such as *cinnamic acid, p-coumaric acid, ferulic acid, caffeic acid, chlorogenic acid, and rosmarinic acid,* belong to this class. These phenolic compounds possess potent antioxidant and anti-inflammatory properties. It's shown benefits for treating diabetics and cholesterol. Hydroxy cinnamic acids are also effective against body weight gain, fat deposition, and dysfunction of the adipocytes because of high-fat diet feeding in animals.

Coffee lovers might love to hear this. Caffeic acid lowered blood glucose, improved insulin resistance, and improved glucose intolerance in high-fat diet-fed mice.[385] Chlorogenic acids are found in coffee as well.

Ferulic acid is one of the most well-studied. It is best known for its skin-protective properties and is used to treat sun damage and reverse the signs of aging, including fine lines and wrinkles. FA has an impressive profile for a wide variety of biological activities such as antioxidant, anti-inflammatory, anti-microbial, anti-allergic, anti-viral, anti-cancer, prevent liver damage, reduce the formation of the blood clot, increase sperm viability, increase blood flow, reduce toxic effects of metal, decrease blood glucose, improve the structure and function of the heart, blood vessels, liver, and kidneys.

Ferulic acid is used as a supplement, which is derived from cereal grains. It also has a high demand for industries such as cosmetics, pharmaceuticals, baking, ice cream, chocolate, and food processing.

FA is found in plants (rice, wheat, oats, and pineapple), grasses, grains, vegetables, flowers, fruits, leaves, beans, seeds of coffee, artichoke, peanut, and nuts. Cell walls of cereal grains and a variety of food plants (pineapple, bananas, spinach, and beetroot). Now you know the secret, and from now on I hope you aren't afraid to eat this type of food anymore. Especially the carbohydrates that some people are afraid to eat. Ferulic acid can also be found in herbal products used in traditional Chinese medicine, such as dong quai (Angelica sinesis), sheng ma (Cimicifuga heracleifolia), and chuan xiong (Ligusticum chuanxiong).

TABLE 4 CONTENT OF FERULIC ACID IN DIFFERENT KNOWN SOURCES.

Source [386]	Ferulic acid (mg./100 g)
Avocado	1.1
Bamboo shoots	243.6
Banana	5.4
Berries	0.25–2.7
Broccoli	4.1
Burdock	7.3–19
Carrot	1.2–2.8
Chinese cabbage	1.4
Coffee	9.1–14.3
Eggplant	7.3–35
Grapefruit	10.7–11.6
Green bean/fresh	1.2
Mizuna	1.4–1.8
Orange	9.2–9.9
Pasta	12

Peanut	8.7
Pickled red beet	39
Plum, dark	1.47
Popcorn	313
Pot grown basil	1.5
Pot grown lettuces	0.19–1.4
Radish	4.6
Red Beet	25
Red Cabbages	6.3–6.5
Rhubarb	2
Rice, brown, long grain parboiled	24
Soyabean	12
Spinach/frozen	7.4
Sugar-beet pulp	800
Sweet corn	42
Tomato	0.29–6
Water dropwort	7.3–34
White wheat bread	8.2

Whole grain oat flakes	25–52
Whole grain rye bread	54

You can see 100 grams of bamboo shoots have 243.6 mg of Ferulic acid. This reminds me of my few favorite Thai dishes I have all the time. For example, red curry with bamboo shoots, bamboo shoots salad, and spicy stir-fried bamboo shoots dishes. Now you know the secret, why Thai women don't get old.

Cinnamic acid is used as a flavor compound in foods and drinks and for its aroma in perfumes and cosmetics. Cinnamic acid is found in the spice cinnamon, which is derived from the bark of trees from the genus Cinnamomum. Cinnamon is well known for its antioxidant, antitumor, antimicrobial, and antimycobacterial properties. [387] Studies also found that cinnamon decreased in levels of fasting blood glucose, total cholesterol, LDL-C, triglyceride levels, and an increase in HDL level. [388] You can also get the benefit of cinnamic acid from other foods such as blueberry, kiwi, cherry, plum, apple, pear, chicory, artichoke, and coffee. [389]

Caffeic acid has many effects on the body, including antioxidant and anti-inflammatory effects. So caffeic acid is often found in skincare regimens.

Caffeic acid, which is unrelated to caffeine. But caffeic acid is found at a tiny level in coffee, at 0.03 mg per 100 ml. But it occurs at high levels in black chokeberry (141 mg per 100 g) and at significant levels in lingonberry (6 mg per 100 g). It is also rich in the South American herb yerba mate (150 mg per 100 g). It is found at a large degree in some herbs in our kitchen, especially thyme, sage and, spearmint (at about 20 mg per

100 g), at significant degrees in spices, Ceylon cinnamon and star anise (at about 22 mg per 100 g), Also in sunflower seeds (8 mg per 100 g), and at modest levels in red wine (1.88 mg per 100 ml). [390] So now you have more ideas to cooperate with the good food for your gut and your body.

Rosmarinic acid, sounds familiar like rosemary, yes you got it right. Rosmarinic acid, named after rosemary, is a polyphenol constituent of many culinary herbs, including rosemary, sage, mint, perilla, basil, salvia, lemon balm, marjoram, and oregano. [391] Many studies reveal that the herbs in your kitchen are so powerful with anti-inflammatory, antioxidant, anti-cancer, anti-tumor, and anti-microbial properties. [392] [393] [394]

Chlorogenic acid plays several important and therapeutic roles such as antioxidant activity, antibacterial, prevent liver damage, cardioprotective, anti-inflammatory, reduce fever, neuroprotective, anti-obesity, antiviral, anti-microbial, anti-hypertension, free radicals scavenger, and a central nervous system (CNS) stimulator.[395] It is found in many foods, including apples, apricots, berries, peaches, pears, plums, avocados, and carrots. It can be found in high amounts in apple juice (6-20 g per 100 g), and green coffee bean (6-9 g per 100 g, so you often see weight loss supplements with green coffee beans. Green coffee beans have 6–9 grams of chlorogenic acid per 100 grams and it's more than roasted coffee beans, which is only 0.2–3 grams per 100 grams of coffee.[396]

3. Lignans

Lignans, which possess a steroid-like chemical structure and are defined as phytoestrogen.

You might have a question. What is phytoestrogen? Phytoestrogen or dietary estrogens are existing compounds found in plants. Estrogen is a hormone released in a woman's body that regulates the menstrual cycle. The body's endocrine system produces this hormone.

At a young age, estrogen plays a part in the development of a woman's breasts, armpit hair, and pubic hair. Estrogen controls a woman's periods until menopause. When you eat plant-based foods that contain phytoestrogen, you may have a similar effect to estrogen produced by the body. For this reason, phytoestrogens are identified as dietary estrogens. There are phytoestrogen supplements but getting these from natural food sources is a better choice and has no side effects.

Health benefits attributed to lignans have included a lowered risk of heart disease, menopausal symptoms, osteoporosis, and breast cancer. Lignans have anti-inflammatory, antioxidant, and antitumor properties. Lignans are found in low concentrations in various seeds, grains, fruits, and vegetables and in higher concentrations in sesame and flax seeds.[397]

Lignan is found in seeds such as flaxseeds, sunflower seeds, almonds, cashew, hazelnut, peanut, chestnut, pecan, walnut, mung beans, white beans, all soy products, miso, tofu, soybeans, edamame, soy flours, etc.

The top 5 highest lignan content of seeds (mg/100g food)

1. Flaxseed (257.6 mg.)
2. Cashew nut (56.33 mg.)
3. Peanut (6.8 mg.)

4. Sunflower seeds (1.52 mg.)

5. Brazil nuts (0.78 mg.)

It's interesting to find out vegetables contain lignan too. Some of them are even higher than cereal grain or beverages, such as coffee and tea.

In the vegetable category, *the brassica family may contain between 185 and 2.321 mg /100 g of lignan, which is higher than cereal grain, fruits, and beverages categories.*

- The highest amount of lignan in the grain category is Rye, whole grain flour (1.46mg.)

- The highest amount of lignan in the fruits category is pear (15.56 mg.), apricot (11.57 mg.), and grapefruit (7.44 mg.)

- The highest amount of lignan in the oil category is sesame seed oil (1294.75 mg.) and sesame seed black oil (1223.3 mg.). Extra virgin olive oil has only 1.08 mg.

You might not eat 100 grams of flaxseed or sesame oil, but every little thing adds up. However, I'm sure you can eat 100 grams and more vegetables. Check out the amazing amount of lignan from vegetables.

Here are the top 10 lignan contents of vegetables (mg/100g food)

1. Broccoli   98.51 mg.

2. Kale   63 mg.

3. Brussel sprouts   50.36 mg.

4. Green bean   22.67 mg.

5. White cabbage   21.51 mg.

6. Sauerkraut   18.3 mg.

7.	Red cabbage	18.1 mg.
8.	Green sweet pepper	12.54 mg.
9.	Cauliflower	9.48 mg.
10.	Red sweet pepper	8.21 mg.

DO YOU KNOW WHY BROCCOLI GOT FAMOUS?

Sweet surprise

It's not only broccoli but also the whole cruciferous family, such as cauliflower, kale, cabbage, brussels sprouts, turnips, kohlrabi, bok choy, and radishes.

From the research, these vegetables contain the sulfur-containing phytochemical glucosinolate, which can be hydrolysed in the human gut to isothiocyanate have anti-cancer properties and protect the development of cancer, heart disease,398 rheumatoid arthritis, type 2 diabetes, obesity, asthma, neurodegenerative diseases, such as Alzheimer's disease. 399 Broccoli sprouts and the sprouts of their family are, in fact, a more concentrated source of these cancer-fighting compounds. 400 How much more? The research mentioned that 3 days old sprouts contain 10-100 times higher levels of glucosinolate than a mature vegetable. 401 I always sprout my broccoli at home. It's very easy and cost-effective.

The best way to get the benefit of isothiocyanate (ITC) and sulforaphane (SF) from broccoli is eating raw, but if your gut can't digest it, stir-fried is not an answer because stir-fried will decrease the properties by 80%.

Here is a trick...

You can boil the broccoli first, then stir-fry it to increase the SF and total ITC concentration by 2.8-2.6 times.402

If you can't eat raw broccoli, but you would love to have the benefit of isothiocyanate sulforaphane. Here is another trick: adding powdered brown mustard to cooked broccoli can increase the sulforaphane over four times more than the cooked broccoli.403

> *If you are in tropical countries and you can't grow broccoli because of the weather, you still can benefit from glucosinolate and isothiocyanate from moringa. 404 Believe me, nature provides you with everything wherever you are in the world.*

Last group is stilbenes.

4. Stilbenes

The subgroups are resveratrol and their cousin, pterostilbene and piceatannol.

The popular resveratrol that people know as the powerful therapeutic option for anti-aging.

What is resveratrol? Resveratrol belongs to a class of polyphenolic compounds called stilbenes. Certain plants produce resveratrol and other stilbenes in response to stress, injury, fungal infection, or ultraviolet (UV) radiation. [405] In the test tube, resveratrol neutralizes free radicals and other oxidants and inhibits low-density lipoprotein (LDL) oxidation. So, if you want to look young and healthy, include the resveratrol-rich food in your daily diet plan.

Resveratrol has been shown to possess many biological activities, which apply to promoting longevity and the prevention and treatment of cancer, cardiovascular disease, and neurodegenerative diseases such as Parkinson's. [406]

HAVE YOU HEARD ABOUT THE FRENCH PARADOX?

The "French Paradox '' — the observation that incidence of coronary heart disease was low in France despite high levels of dietary saturated fat and cigarette smoking — led to the idea that regular consumption of red wine might provide additional protection from cardiovascular disease. However, the result showed that moderate alcohol intake does not prevent coronary heart disease. [407] Red wine contains variable and low concentrations of resveratrol and higher concentrations of flavonoids like procyanidins. These polyphenolic compounds have displayed antioxidant, anti-inflammatory properties, and other protective effects on the formation of plaques in arteries. So, it's excellent for your heart health.

How much resveratrol is in 5 oz. of wine? It's only 0.2-0.5 mg. However, if you want to get a little resveratrol from wine, Pinot Noir gives a higher number than other types of wine.[408]

Resveratrol is a natural phenol and phytoalexin, produced by 72 different plant species, especially grapevines, pines, and legumes. It is also present in itadori tea (or Japanese knotweed), peanuts, soybeans, cacao, berries, grapes, and pomegranates. Itadori tea shows that they contain trans-resveratrol glucosides. In contrast, red wines are a source of taglycones cis- and trans-resveratrol. While peanuts and grapes contain low levels of the stilbenes.[409]

Most resveratrol supplements available in the US contain extracts of the root of Polygonum cuspidatum, also known as Fallopia japonica, Japanese knotweed, or Hu Zhang.

IS IT WORTH DRINKING RED WINE FOR RESVERATROL?

Compare the resveratrol in 5 oz. red wine is 0.5 mg, 1 cup (180 g) boiled peanut is 0.32 mg, and 1 cup (160 g) red grapes is 0.24 mg.

Another research of resveratrol in mulberry, jamun, grapes and, jackfruit. Mulberry whole fruit extracts showed the highest concentration of resveratrol 50.61 µg g−1 followed by Jamun seed extracts and their pulp and skin extracts is 34.87 - 11.19 µg g–1 and grapes seed extracts their pulp and skin extracts is 5.89- 1.44 µg g–1. However, Grape seed extracts were found to have more phenolic content when compared to other extracts analyzed.

Research in Europe for Stilbenes - resveratrol in food and beverage.[410]

Check table 5 for detail

TABLE 5 RESVERATROL IN FOOD

Food & Beverage	Type	Mean content	Note
Wines - Berry wines	Fox grape, red wine	0.25 mg/100 ml	
	Fox grape, white wine	0.01 mg/100 ml	
	Muscadine grape, red wine	3.02 mg/100 ml	
Wines - Grape wines	Wine [Red]	0.27 mg/100 ml	Brazilian wine - Merlot 2002 Giacomin in tank 2.78 mg/100 ml
	Wine [Rosé]	0.12 mg/100 ml	
	Wine [White]	0.04 mg/100 ml	
Wines - Sparkling wines	Champagne	9.00e-03 mg/100 ml	

Cocoa - Chocolate	Chocolate, dark	0.04 mg/100 g FW	
Fruits - Berries	Bilberry, raw	0.67 mg/100 g FW	
	European cranberry	1.92 mg/100 g FW	
	Grape [Black]	0.15 mg/100 g FW	
	Grape [Green]	0.02 mg/100 g FW	
	Lingonberry, raw	3.00 mg/100 g FW	
	Redcurrant, raw	1.57 mg/100 g FW	
	Strawberry, raw	0.35 mg/100 g FW	
Nuts	Peanut	0.08 mg/100 g FW	Runner peanuts has the highest score. 1.12 mg/100 g FW
	Peanut, dehulled	0.07 mg/100 g FW	
	Peanut, dehulled, roasted	0.02 mg/100 g FW	
	Pistachio, dehulled	0.11 mg/100 g FW	

FW= Fresh weight

Wine from different countries and regions gives different numbers of resveratrol. According to this research, it surprised me that Brazilian wine has more resveratrol than wine from France. Here are the top 3 Brazilian wines:

1. 2.78 mg/100 ml Brazilian wine - Merlot 2002 Giacomin in tank

2. 2.67 mg/100 ml Brazilian wine - Merlot 2002 Giacomin commercial

3. 2.50 mg/100 ml Brazilian wine - Merlot 2003 micro-winemaking

Sweet surprise

Papaya seeds have polyphenol too. So next time you eat papaya, don't throw away the seeds of youth. You can dry them and eat dry seeds for the next 48 hours, or you can also put them in the blender and add them to your food like black pepper. I also use it for a papaya dressing recipe.

Christopher Columbus called papaya "the fruit of the angels." Papaya seeds contain polyphenols, flavonoids, and the antioxidant capacity of methanol extracts (ME) and hexane extracts (HE). 411 The antioxidants in papaya fruit and seeds and their high fiber have an abundance of unique qualities that promote the detox process, the kidney detox. The protein-rich papaya seeds contain glycine and proline, 412 the essential amino acids that boost your collagen production. The papain, an active enzyme in papaya seeds and raw papaya, helps for skin generation and repair so you can have a more youthful glow, as the studied in papain use for their glycosides, phenolic acids, such as caffeic acid and ferulic acid. A new study in 2021 revealed that papayas contain high amounts of natural antioxidants that can be found in their leaves, fruits, and seeds. It contains various chemical compounds that show significant antioxidant properties, including caffeic acid, myricetin, rutin, quercetin, α-tocopherol, papain, benzyl isothiocyanate (BiTC), and kaempferol. Therefore, it can counteract pro-oxidants via several signaling pathways that either promote the expression of antioxidant enzymes or reduce ROS production.

Oxidative stress occurs because of excessive ROS production, which will cause oxidative damage to tissues. Consequence effects of oxidative stress have known to cause inflammation, leading to the development

of various health conditions, including Alzheimer's Disease (AD), rheumatoid disease, cardiovascular diseases (CVDs), cancers, cataracts, as well as cosmetic issues, such as the formation of wrinkles and loss of elasticity of the skin. Flavonoids in papaya are kaempferol, myricetin, quercetin, and their glycosides, phenolic acids, such as caffeic acid and ferulic acid, are the key ROS suppressors and antioxidants that displayed radical scavenging and metal chelating potential. Caffeic acid and rutin were detected and proposed to be the main anti-skin aging components. 413 Now you know the powerful tropical beauty. From now on, don't throw away any part of "the fruit of the angels".

The richest sources of polyphenols were various spices and dried herbs, cocoa products, some darkly colored berries, some seeds (flaxseed) and nuts (chestnut, hazelnut), and some vegetables, including olive and globe artichoke heads. Wine doesn't have as many polyphenols as people think.

TABLE 6 POLYPHENOL CONTENT IN THE TOP 30 RICHEST FOODS

(mg per 100 g or mg per 100 ml) [414]

Food	Polyphenol content
1. Cloves	15 188
2. Peppermint, dried	11 960
3. Star anise	5460
4. Cocoa powder	3448
5. Mexican oregano, dried	2319
6. Celery seed Seasonings	2094
7. Black chokeberry	1756
8. Dark chocolate	1664
9. Flaxseed meal	1528
10. Black elderberry	1359
11. Chestnut	1215
12. Common sage, dried	1207
13. Rosemary, dried	1018
14. Spearmint, dried	956
15. Common thyme, dried	878
16. Lowbush blueberry	836
17. Blackcurrant	758
18. Capers	654
19. Black olive	569
20. Highbush blueberry	560
21. Hazelnut	495

22. Pecan nut	493
23. Soy flour	466
24. Plum	377
25. Green olive	346
26. Sweet basil, dried	322
27. Curry, powder	285
28. Sweet cherry	274
29. Globe artichoke heads	260
30. Blackberry	260

Some foods, such as spices and herbs, can be rich in polyphenols, but the amount consumed is low. Therefore, it is also important to estimate the number of polyphenols in a serving (Table 7).

TABLE 7 TOP 30 POLYPHENOL AND ANTIOXIDANT CONTENTS

(mg per serving) [415]

Food	Food group	Serving a (g)	Polyphenols b		Polyphenols AE b		Antioxidants c	
			Content	Rank	Content	Rank	Content	Rank
Black elderberry	Fruits	145d	1956	1	1196	2	2808	1
Black chokeberry	Fruits	145d	1595	2	1114	1	2523	2
Blackcurrant	Fruits	145d	1092	3	689	4	1182	5
Highbush blueberry	Fruits	145d	806	4	425	5	321	14
Globe artichoke heads	Vegetables	168	436	5	259	8	1918	3
Coffee, filter	Non-alcoholic beverages	190	408	6	209	13	507	11
Lowbush blueberry	Fruits	145d	395	7	714	3	678	8

Sweet cherry	Fruits	145d	394	8	209	14	249	20
Strawberry	Fruits	166d	390	9	340	6	480	12
Blackberry	Fruits	144d	374	10	260	9	821	6
Plum	Fruits	85	320	11	242	11	349	13
Red raspberry	Fruits	144	310	12	154	17	213	22
Flaxseed meal	Seeds	20e	306f	13	244f	10	—	—
Dark chocolate	Cocoa products	17	283	14	275	7	316	15
Chestnut	Seeds	19	230	15	231	12	524	10
Black tea	Non-alcoholic beverages	195	197	16	175	15	204	23
Green tea	Non-alcoholic beverages	195	173	17	164	16	121	31
Pure apple juice	Non-alcoholic beverages	248	168	18	151	18	84	38

Apple	Fruits	110	149	19	147	19	221	21
Whole grain rye bread	Cereals	120	146f	20	146f	20	—	—
Hazelnut	Seeds	28e	138	21	138	21	192	24
Red wine	Alcoholic beverages	125	126	22	117	23	269	19
Soy yogurt	Seeds	125	105	23	53	28	—	—
Cocoa powder	Cocoa products	3	103	24	99	25	33	46
Pure pomegranate juice	Non-alcoholic beverages	150	99	25	50	31	306	16
Soy flour	Seeds	20e	93	26	53	29	—	—
Black grape	Fruits	54	91	27	113	24	92	36
Black olive	Vegetables	15	85	28	48	32	17	56
Pure grapefruit juice	Non-alcoholic beverages	150	79	29	39	37	82	39

Pure blood orange juice	Non-alcoholic beverages	154	71	30	31	42	111	33

1. Abbreviation: AE, (polyphenols as) aglycone equivalents.

2. a From the Food Standards Agency, UK (Food Standards Agency, 2002), except for values marked with a superscript.

3. b Sum of individual polyphenols determined by reverse-phase high-performance liquid chromatography (HPLC) and proanthocyanidins oligomers determined by direct-phase HPLC.

4. c Determined by the Folin assay.

Now you learn about the polyphenol in different foods. So, it's not only red wine, grapes, and berries like most people think. People in Asia and in the tropics with tropical climates do not have easy access to berries and grapes, or they don't drink wine at all. They still get the benefit of polyphenols from many other food sources.

Please note that polyphenol supplements are not the best choice. It's better to get from a food source. *Research in 2018 mentioned that some harmful effects had been reported from polyphenol intake.* Adverse outcomes have been documented from polyphenolic botanical extracts in beverages, especially for individuals with a degenerative disease, high blood pressure, thyroid disease, epilepsy, or heart disease that are more harmful than helpful. [416]

You know all the polyphenol-rich foods that can boost your gut microbiota. Remember, once you give them food, they will multiply and thrive. Then you will get the benefit of SCFs, and soon you will feel better from inside out, starting from your gut, your brain, and all body functions, including your waistline and immunity.

TO-DO-LIST

1. Pick your top 10 fruits and vegetables.

2. Check it out if your favorite fruits and vegetables have 7 colors, like a rainbow. If yes, perfect, but if not, try to add some to complete your rainbow food. Remember, your gut microbiome loves varieties of fiber, so try to mix and match for your own benefit.

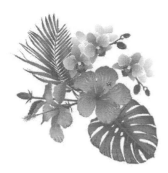

CHAPTER 8

BONUS FOR YOU

BONUS # 1. EXERCISE AS A TOOL TO ACCELERATE YOUR RESULTS

In this department, I want to tell you-you are in good hands since I've been a certified personal trainer for over 15 years, and I also had proved that I changed my body composition as I have won a bodybuilding show in Northern California, and I lost 20 pounds in 100 days even before I became a certified personal trainer. However, when I lost weight and maintained my weight after my accident, I didn't do a lot of exercise at all. So, I want to tell you that exercise is not a priority, but the food you take in every day is. If you can exercise to your full potential, go for it, but if you can't do it, just like me. You can reach your weight loss goal as fast as other people too. The key is to keep moving. Not for calorie deficit but for hormone balance and brain chemistry, as I mentioned in chapters 3 and 4.

If your goal is losing 10 pounds or more, overcoming sugar addiction, or lowering your HbA1C level. You will benefit from exercise since it will help to speed up your results, and as you learned from chapter 3, exercise or physical activities can help you boost the brain chemistry, dopamine, and serotonin. A study in 2021 showed that physical exercise is a tool to help the immune system against COVID-19.
[417]

If you can exercise, here is the way to do it.

Exercise only 30 minutes for 4 days/ week

I understand time is valuable, especially for us in our 40s, 50s, and 60s, because we are at the age that is involved with building the career. You might be at your peak time, or you have family and children to take care of. So, time for people in their 40s and 50 might be limited. I understand, and I got you covered.

You will do 2 types of exercise for 30 minutes/ day and only 4 days per week

1. Weight training
2. High-Intensity Interval Training (HIIT)

Weight training

or resistance training will help you to burn more calories since it helps you to build muscle mass, so you will burn more calories even when you do nothing.

Have you heard about BMR and RMR?

BMR (Basal Metabolic Rate) is an estimate of how many calories you would burn if you were to do nothing but rest for 24 hours. It represents the minimum amount of energy needed to keep your body functioning, including breathing and keeping your heart beating.

RMR (Resting metabolic rate) is, also known as Resting Energy Expenditure (REE), is the energy required to keep your body functioning at rest. It's slightly different from BMR. There are many factors that can affect your RMR. Muscle Mass is one of those factors. The more muscles you have, the higher your Resting Metabolic Rate is.

I might write another book for all the details for weight training for women and men over 40 because the training is slightly different from when you are in your 20 or 30. Training for men and women is a little bit different, too. For now, let's keep these few important things as follows.

- Warm-up, but do not stretch before your weight training session. Warming up might be 5 minutes walking, or warm up with any cardio machine you like if you are in the gym, then swing your arms and your legs. For someone who has been lifting for a while, the warm-up might be a lighter weight of the first exercise of the body part, either upper body or lower body.

- Work on bigger muscles before small muscles. For example, you will want to work on your chest before your triceps.

- If you do a full-body workout, I recommend starting from the upper back, legs (mainly squat, no isolation), chest, shoulders, keep arms, and abdominal last.

- Cool down. Now you can enjoy stretching at the end of your workout.

- If you have time and energy after your 30 minutes of weight training, you can go for a walk or do cardio on any cardio machine at low - medium intensity. It's easy to fit in for busy people. After 30 minutes of lifting weight, you just walk home, bike home, take your dog for a walk or do gardening.

High-intensity interval training (HIIT)

HIIT is simply alternating short bursts of intense activity with longer intervals of less intense activity. The range of work and recovery for each interval is 15 seconds up to 2-3 minutes in duration (depending on the ratio of work-to-recovery used). Interval training not only helps you to burn more body fat and calories 24 hours after your workout but also significantly increases growth hormone (GH)[418] and Brain-derived neurotrophic factor(BDNF), [419] which is a brain-promoting neurotrophic factor. You can also get the benefit of interval training with heart health and circulation.

Growth hormones help you lose weight

Do you remember I mentioned that growth hormones are one of the hormones that can help you lose weight? Now I can tell you a little bit more. Growth hormones are antidiabetics. The effects of GH on systemic glycemic control are complex partly because of its indirect effects via insulin-like growth factor 1 (IGF-1), which has glucose-lowering effects similar to insulin. GH showed markedly increased gluconeogenesis activity in the liver and kidney. GH stimulates lipolysis via activation of the hormone-sensitive lipase, primarily in the visceral adipose tissue, which results in free fatty acid (FFA) flux from adipose tissue to circulation. [420]After you hear this from me, you might think I can take growth hormones. Hold on! Something that is not natural always has a side effect. If you take growth hormones, it will work for a short time period, and your body won't produce on its own because your body thinks they don't need to do the job while they have a supply from somewhere else. Your body is smart!

How to do the correct interval training

You can do any activity, such as walking, running, swimming, hiking, kickboxing, jumping, biking, burpee, stairs climbing, or any exercise on any cardio machine. The goal is to bring your heart rate up as close as you can to your maximum heart rate. In the studies, high-intensity aerobic interval training refers to walking or running intensity at bouts of 85%-90% of peak oxygen uptake or 90%-95% of peak heart rate, separated by 2-3 minutes of active recovery at approximately 60%-70% of peak heart rate.[421]

Here's the formula: 220 - your age = your maximal heart rate (MHR). I'm 46; my maximum heart is 220-46= 174 beats per minute(bpm)

My 85% MHR is 148

My 95% MHR is 165

My 60% MHR is 104

My 70% MHR is 122

I will go for a short and high intensity with my MHR 148 - 165 bpm. And recovery with MHR 104-122 bpm. The more fit you are, you will get to the recovery zone fast. So, if your MHR gets to 70% in 60 seconds, then you should work upon your intensity again. But if it takes you to get to your 70% for 2 minutes, it's ok. Everyone is different. In the beginning, you might want to monitor your heart rate with a watch or cardio machine your handhold and track your heart rate. But if you don't have access to one, just go as fast as you can like our ancestors ran while the tiger tried to catch them and slow down when they found a bush to hide or climb to a nice tree for safety.

Women and men can do HIIT a little differently for the maximum result. For women, I would recommend doing 30 seconds of peak maximum heart rate of 85% - 95% (depending on how fit you are) and recovery for 90 seconds or if you check your heart rate at approximately 60%-70%. Men would benefit from short bursts and longer rest. I would recommend 15-20 seconds go as fast as you can, then rest for 2-3 minutes. You will come back with a full recovery and go strong.

This is how you do it.

- 5 minutes warm-up on a cardio machine or any activity that you choose.

- Start at 6 minutes go as fast as you can for a short time period

- Followed by a resting period

- Do the fast and short one again until 24 minutes of the total time.

- Then cool down for 5 minutes

- Here is an example: I will do a 30/90 interval. I will reach a peak at all even numbers in 24 minutes. (6,8,10,12,14,16,18,20,22,24) So you will get the 10 cycles. For men, you can do super short but explode for 15-20seconds, then rest for a longer period. It doesn't matter how many cycles you get. The most important thing is you get to the 85%-95% MHR, then recover and go back strong to get 85%-95% MHR again in 20 minutes. Remember, you warm up 5 minutes or 10 minutes if you want to and cool down for 5 minutes, then you are done with a short but sweet workout.

So, if you have a time limit, you can do these 30 minutes exercises for 4 days per week whenever you have more time to do activities outdoors, for example, hiking, swimming, walking, or biking. The great time and enjoyment will help to boost your brain chemistry and also help for hormone balance.

BONUS # 2. A SOLUTION FOR SOMEONE WHO CAN'T EXERCISE

If you can't exercise because you are injured, have chronic pain, or just don't have time. I have some tips for you since I also got in an accident in 2017, and it became a chronic pain. However, I can still manage my weight. By the way, in the picture you saw on the cover, I didn't do much exercise, so it's no weight training and zero-time HIIT.

Stay tuned. I'm going to share my secret with you.

Have you heard about the blue zone? People live to a healthy 100 in 5 different places in the world; Ikaria in Greece, Sardinia in Italy, Okinawa in Japan, Nicoya Peninsula in Costa Rica and Loma Linda in California, USA.

> The most important part of longevity, healthy and no weight gain are 3 keys essential factors.
>
> 1. Food
>
> 2. Keep moving
>
> 3. Less stress

Look back to chapter 3. I mentioned the hormones that make you gain weight and store fat are insulin and cortisol or stress hormones.

People who live in the blue zone do not go for exercise or the gym, but they keep moving. They have less stress. Therefore, they have the hormone harmony with their body. They eat food from their backyard, the local source, and food are from the mother of earth, but not processed food from the manufacturer where we found them in the box and container. They eat whole-food plant-based, which is different than vegetarian or vegan. Sometimes they eat fish, meat, or poultry, and those are from local, not farm-raised, no antibacterial to the animal they eat. But you know what, they do not eat meat and poultry often.

My secret for weight loss, apart from the food mentioned in chapters 4,5,6,7 and keeping hormones balanced, I do the following instead of "exercise."

1. Keep moving

You might have physical limitations or injuries, but you can move. So, move the way you can. Most people with lower back and lower body injuries can move in the water. So go into the water and move. You don't need to swim. Just move the way you can in the water, which has resistance, so now you move every part of your body against the resistance. You can move freely with no pain or less for someone.

The secret is that you must do it in the morning, so you get MORNING Sunlight which reinforces your natural circadian rhythms. The power of the sun will help to boost your serotonin and dopamine.

Your body's circadian systems manufacture many of your biological processes, including your hormones, hunger, energy levels, and body temperature.

Most people like to be in the water because it's soothing. I live in Hawaii so I can go to the ocean. You can go to a lake, river or pool, whatever you can. Apart from moving, you also get less stress. Now you also control your hormone cortisol which can trigger fat storage.

If you can't get into the water for any reason. You just move the way you can. Here is an idea; walking, tai chi, yoga, stretching, gardening, doing things in your backyard, or even sitting down and using exercising resistance bands (In case you can't stand or move much). <u>But remember</u>

to keep moving in the morning sun and without sunglasses. You know our ancestors did not have sunglasses.

2. Sit in a sauna

If you can move or not move, you can sit or lie down in the sauna because once you sit in there, your heart will beat faster, just like you do low-intensity cardio exercise. Sauna has so many benefits, such as.

- Increase growth hormone. [422] [423]

- Increase testosterone hormone.

- Decrease cortisol, therefore, reduces stress levels and makes you feel good afterward. [424] [425]

- Increase longevity

- Promotes heart health with a better cardiovascular and circulatory function.[426]

- Lower blood pressure [427]

- Help With Detoxification through the skin; the body's largest organ. [428]

- Improve Insulin Sensitivity. [429]

- Help with fat loss. The sauna improves insulin sensitivity, helps clear glucose from the blood, stimulates detoxification, and promotes growth hormone levels, so saunas can indirectly encourage fat loss.

- Help prevent muscle breakdown and increase the size of muscles (Hypertrophy) [430] [431]

- Increases Endurance Performance. [432] [433]

- Boost Immunity. [434] [435]

- Help Reduce Pain. [436] [437] [438]

- Increases the growth of new brain cells since the brain-derived neurotrophic factor (BDNF) increases when the body is exposed to heat stress. [439]

- Increase autophagy. Autophagy is the body's way of cleaning out damaged cells in order to regenerate newer and healthier cells. [440] [441]

- Help you have a good night's sleep.

3. Intermittent fasting

I did 16/8 intermittent fasting to achieve my weight loss goal and health while I couldn't exercise as I used to. Intermittent fasting has so many benefits to you, such as can reduce insulin resistance, dropping your risk for type 2 diabetes, can cut down oxidative stress and inflammation in the body, can help you lose weight and visceral fat, boosting growth hormones, enhancing autophagy (or cellular repair), increase levels of a brain-derived neurotrophic factor (BDNF). [442] [443] [444] [445] [446] [447] [448] [449] And if this is not cool enough. I want to tell you that intermittent fasting can turn your white fat into brown fat and help everybody lose belly fat and forget about insulin resistance and metabolic x syndrome. This might be another book to share with you because not all intermittent fasting can do that trick.

How I did it's so simple. I woke up, drank lemon water with apple cider vinegar, drank green tea, and then went to the ocean for swimming, moving, or walking, but the most important thing was soaking in the morning sun. I will have my first meal at noon, and the next one is around 4 pm. Like a small snack before going for an evening walk with my dog. I will have my dinner around 7:00 pm. - 8:00 pm. After that, I will go to the sauna. I tried to go to the sauna every night, but if I miss it some night, it's not a big deal. I tried to do a body scrub 1-2/times per week between my sauna or after the sauna. It will help with blood circulation and clean the biggest organ, the skin. Remember, you do the detox; you clean from the inside out. Yes, you cleanse your liver, kidney, and gut. But how about skin?

BONUS # 3. TAKING CARE OF YOUR LARGEST ORGAN

This chapter is a bonus. Yes, it's a real bonus for you. I 'm sharing my secret ingredients of beauty & youthfulness with you. Ladies, you will love my recipes, and gentlemen, I want to tell you if you do it, your body will say thank you. Skin is your largest organ, and it's essential to take care of it, even though you take care from the inside out. Radiant skin shows how you take good care of your overall health. The skin treatment is not only for women. Whoever has skin, you got to give them some treatment if you want them to look good and feel great.

I didn't tell you before that I'm also a licensed massage therapist, and I ran a business in Hawaii for a while. So, I know a few of the best natural treatments. It would be best if you didn't use a store-bought for your skin treatment during your detox because you don't want a chemical to mix in while you want to get rid of it.

Here are a few recipes for body treatment

<u>Kona coffee rub (Cellulite buster)</u>

- 2 cups coarsely ground Kona coffee (or use other coffee but choose an organic coffee)
- ½ cup raw sugar
- 3 Tbsp olive oil

Mix ingredients well. Take a hot shower (or after a sauna) to moisten the skin and open pores. Using a wide, circular motion, rub coffee exfoliant on your body with firm, even pressure. Rinse well.

Sweet body scrubs

- ½ cup brown sugar

- Juice ½ orange

- 1 Tbsp vitamin E oil

- Optional: 3-5 drops doTERRA essential oil (wild orange, grapefruit, citrus bloom, or tangerine)

Mix all ingredients. Apply after a hot shower, sauna, or bath. Apply the mixture with a gentle circular motion. Rinse and enjoy.

You can check out my website: my.doterra.com/Triya

Macadamia cleansing grains

- 2 cup oatmeal

- ½ cup unsalted macadamia nuts

- 2 Tbsp dried rose petals

- 2 Tbsp dried lavender flowers

- Warm water (enough to make a paste)

- (optional) ½ tsp. Almond oil.

Finely grind each dry ingredient in separate batches. Mix well and store in a covered container in a cool, dry place. To use, mix 1 heaping teaspoon of cleansing grains with enough warm water to make a creamy paste. If you have dry skin, add almond oil. Gently massage the mixture onto your skin. Rinse with warm water.

The facial treatment

I have a few recipes for you. DIY from natural ingredients while you detox your internal organs, so please do not put chemicals on your skin. Feel free to ask or share the recipes in the Facebook community. It's fun to do it together.

Anti-Aging Spirulina Face Mask

- 1 tablespoon spirulina

- 1 tablespoon sweet almond oil or castor oil

- 2 drops vitamin E oil

Skin for 40+ needs lots of moisture and antioxidants, and this mask provides both. It plumps up the skin, coats it in a layer of healing, nourishing oils, and protects it from free radicals.

Mix all the ingredients well together. Once you get a smooth paste, apply it to your face. Leave it on for 15–20 minutes. Wash the mask off and apply your moisturizer while your skin is still damp to lock in the moisture.

Rejuvenate Tropical Face Mask

- 1 tablespoon pineapple puree

- 1 tablespoon papaya puree

- 2 teaspoons jojoba oil

Pineapple and papaya are a powerful combination that can revive your skin, rejuvenate it, and make it smooth and radiant in no time. Jojoba oil has a quality that our skin easily absorbs. It is nourishing perfect for all skin types.

Mix all the ingredients well together. Apply the paste to your face in a thick, even layer. Take 5 minutes to massage the mask into your skin, then leave the mask on for 5 more minutes.

Rinse it off using lukewarm water. Apply a lightweight face moisturizer while your skin is still damp to lock in the moisture and keep your skin well-hydrated and nourished for longer.

Mango glow & flawless skin

- 2 Tbsp. mango

- 1 Tbsp. Oatmeal finely powdered.

- 1 Tbsp. Almond finely powdered.

- 1 Tbsp. coconut cream (or yogurt)

- Distilled water or mineral water (as needed: optional)

Mangoes are loaded with beta-carotene, polyphenol, and vitamin A, which helps your skin get back its natural glow and radiance. It promotes collagen production, keeps the skin wrinkle-free, and slows down premature aging.

Blend all ingredients until the mixture is creamy. (If too runny, add more oatmeal.) Apply on your face and neck. Scrub it off after 15 minutes and rinse with warm water. Apply moisturizer while your skin is still damp. You can also apply rosehip oil or other natural oil before going to bed.

I hope you love the recipes and have a pleasant time doing it while you are on the 21 days sugar detox program. Sometimes you might wonder, so how about going to a spa and getting a facial done? Oh yes, talking about a spa. You might think about massage too. Who doesn't love a massage? Next, I would like to share an idea for reward systems with you, and you might get excited about my reward system.

BONUS # 4. REWARD SYSTEM

You have heard about the reward system with children. Did you know rewarding yourself is extremely beneficial for adults!? A reward is required for any goal or habit! Whether you have a weight loss goal or just want to change a habit of living without sugar and refined carbohydrate.

Reward system = Motivation

Know your weakness and turn it into your strength, then reward yourself.

Know what your bad habit is and make it a good one, then reward yourself.

For example,

- It's difficult for me to stop drinking wine, so once I stopped drinking, I gave myself 5 points.

- It's difficult for me to stop eating after 8:00 pm., so once I stop eating after 8:00 pm. I gave myself 5 points.

- It's difficult for me to stop eating potato chips, so once I stopped eating, I gave myself 5 points.

- It's difficult for me to go to bed early, so once I go to bed early, I gave myself 5 points.

I would recommend you set your reward system to motivate and improve whatever you wish in your life. Right now, you do sugar detox, so it's perfect for you to set the reward system. Once you do this, you will be proud of yourself. You can use the points and exchange to be money, and money can exchange to be an activity, treatment, or an object unrelated to food & drink. For example, you want a facial treatment, a 1-hour massage, a new workout clothes, a trip to a tropical island, and everything in the universe that you wish.

Sweet Surprise

Visualization is truly remarkable.

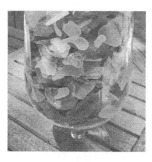

I will put on points in the clear jar or glasses that I can see every day. I use sea glass because I love the color and get it when I walk on the beach. You can use marble, coins, seashell, coffee beans, or anything you want in the jar, and you will see them every day.

At the end of 21 days, sugar detox. You will have your points to appreciate whatever you desire! Don't forget to share in the Facebook community.

TO-DO-LIST

Preparation for success

Read bonus 1-4, what do you need to prep for your situation.

For example, you need to buy exercising resistance bands, jojoba oil, or vitamin E oil.

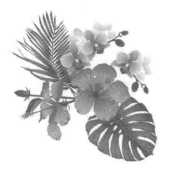

CHAPTER 9

WHAT IS IN AND WHAT IS OUT IN 21 DAYS SUGAR DETOX

1. Give up sugar

Of course, that is what this book is all about. Please don't laugh. This is a recap for you.

1.1 Get rid of any food that has sugar and fructose. Check chapter 2 Fifty-six names of sugar (You may keep brown sugar and honey for body and facial treatment). Check for more updates in the Facebook community. We might have more sugar names in the future.

1.2 Do not buy any food that has those fifty-six names of sugar in it. Exceptional for chocolate. In these 21 days of sugar detox, you can have chocolate and I have some recipes for you, but if you don't want to make it and you can't find anything that tastes good with stevia or monk fruit, you may have real sugar in the ingredients, but not the first ingredients. Sugar content shouldn't be over 10 grams per serving. If you follow the menu plan, you won't consume more sugar than the daily limit. So, you are good to go with chocolate with less than 10 grams per serving. If you find any chocolate you like, please share it with friends in the Facebook community.

1.3 Sugar substitutes

Greenlight: Nutritive sweeteners or sugar alcohol are good (sorbitol, xylitol, mannitol, erythritol, isomalt, and lactitol). Everything is good except the maltitol.

Nonnutritive sweeteners, natural sweeteners: Monk fruit extract, licorice, Thaumatin are good. Oh! Also, yacon syrup. Because it comes from the yacon root.

Yellow light: Stevia extract may affect the gut microbiome, but it's still ok in small amounts.

Red light: Nonnutritive sweeteners, synthetic sweeteners (acesulfame K, aspartame, cyclamate, saccharin, neotame, advantame, sucralose), everything that FDA approved that are not good for your body systems and the gut microbiome.

2. Fat and oil

Greenlight: Extra virgin olive oil, unrefined coconut oil, sesame oil, avocado fruit (but not avocado oil), all nuts and seeds, all nut kinds of butter (natural and no sugar added)

Yellow light: Avocado oil, ghee, butter.

Red light: All vegetable oils, and animal fat

3. Protein source

These 21 days sugar detox is vegan and vegetarian friendly.

Greenlight: All plant-based proteins, fish (wild-caught) and seafood (wild-caught, local only, no farm-raised import from Asia), all seaweed, and all the sea vegetables.

Aonori, Arame, Badderlocks, Dulse, Nori, Guso/Eucheuma, Hijiki, Irish Moss, Kombu, Oarweed, Ogonori, Sea Grapes, Sea Lettuce, Wakame

Red meat (Beef and bison only beef grass-fed grass-finished, wild game), eggs (Pasture-Raised eggs and organic pasture-raised eggs)

Yellow light: All Organic free-range chicken products, organic chicken sausage (no preservative & no MSG), pork (Only raised without antibiotics)

Red light: Turkey, pork, chicken, sausages (except mentioned in yellow light), red meat and egg (except mentioned in green light).

4. Carbohydrates

4.1 Fruits

<u>Greenlight</u>: All fruits except bananas.

<u>Yellow light:</u> Ripe banana (Ripe banana is high in sucrose & glucose. Everyone will have a different reaction to ripe bananas. The recipes banana & avocado together is ok)

*Note: follow the recipes and note on meal menu

<u>Red light</u>: None

4.2 Vegetables

<u>Greenlight</u>: All vegetables

<u>Yellow light</u>: Some starchy vegetables for a non-vegetarian meal (follow the menu plan)

<u>Red light</u>: None

4.3 Starch & grains

<u>Greenlight:</u> All grains & starch for vegetarian meal menu

<u>Yellow light</u>: (non-vegetarian menu plan) some grains & starch will be limited. (Follow the menu plan), sourdough bread.

<u>Red light:</u> All ultra-processed food, sweet or savory packaged snacks, mass-produced packaged; bread and buns, cookies (biscuits), pastries, cakes, and cake mixes; breakfast 'cereals', 'cereal', pre-made, and white rice.

5. Beverage

<u>Greenlight</u>: filter water, mineral water, sparkling mineral water, green tea, black tea, white tea, herbal tea, oolong tea, rooibos tea, posted-fermented tea (Pu-erh tea), decaf coffee (swiss water process only)

<u>Yellow light:</u>

1. organic coffee (only 1 cup/ day the first week, 1-2 cups/day week 2 and 3)

2. A bottle of commercial kombucha drink (only 1 serving if sugar is less than 7 g/serving, if sugar is more than 7g/serving, you can have less and do your math)

3. Red wine (None for week 1 but weeks 2 & 3 is ok if you can keep 1 serving for women and 2 servings for men. If you know yourself that you can't stop after finishing your daily serving. Do not have red wine at all during the detox)

4. Coconut water, it's ok to add in a smoothie.

Red light:

1. Tap water, purified water, all water (except mentioned in green light)

2. Water in plastic bottle

3. Soda

4. Energy drinks

5. All juice

6. A regular decaf coffee

7. All alcohol (except red wine)

8. All drinks that are not mentioned in green light and yellow light.

6. Condiment & Spice

Greenlight: All spices with no salt added, all fresh & dry spices & herbs.

soy products - choose only organic, i.e., organic tamari, organic soy sauce, organic miso, organic Nama shoyu.

Iodine salt, Sea salt (Naturally contains iodine.), pink Himalayan salt (not usually iodized), black Himalayan salt (not usually iodized)

<u>Red light:</u> All sauce and any products with MSG, sauce or condiment contain vegetable oils

Superfood

Moringa, spirulina, maca, curcumin, and turmeric.

Supplement

Must have list:

1. Omega 3

    I recommend omega-3 from algae oil. (Take only the day you do not consume omega-3 from food).

2. Milk thistle 250 mg. Take 1 capsule twice a day during your 21 days detox.

3. Trace mineral drops.

Good to have list:

1. Probiotic supplement, look for multi-strain. Everyone is different. During the 21 days of sugar detox, you will have prebiotic and probiotics from food. However, some of you might need extra help.

2. Vitamin D 3 (If you don't get enough sun) First choice, you get vitamin D from the sun for at least 45 minutes to 1 hour each day or get it from a food source. If during winter or bad weather you don't get enough sun, then you should take vitamin D. Remember, vitamin D is not a vitamin but a hormone.

    Other supplements, you don't need, if you get enough from food. Check chapter 4 if you are lacking anything. I would recommend getting all of them from a food source.

    I hope you discover favorable information and adapt it for your own health and wellness. You may do detox 1 to 3 times a year. I like to do it before New Year, early spring (40 days lent), and early fall season. You can use the recipes from week 2 and 3 all year round.

Every time you go to the grocery store, you can use it as a reference. Now you know what is good for your gut, brain, and body. After finishing this book, you know the reason why you choose healthy food and lifestyle. You know what food you should look for when you go to the grocery store, and no one can fool you for their products for weight loss. You have the key to weight loss, longevity, and overcoming sugar and refined carb cravings, and addiction. Now you can use your tools.

For some of you who want to get the results as soon as possible, or you have insulin resistance, low HDL and high triglyceride, pre-diabetes, high blood pressure or you need extra assistance in your health and wellness journey. Please feel free to contact me for one-on-one coaching. You can reach me at Triya@Alohatriya.com

I hope you find balance, harmony, and joy in your journey. Feel free to join me in the Facebook group and I hope to see you with a big smile!

"Life is in your hand. Choose the right choice

and travel in the right way...

-Mery Anthony-

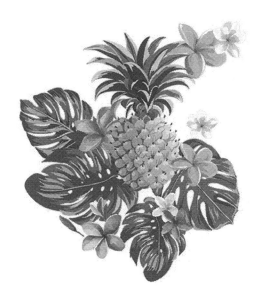

If you enjoyed this book !

You found useful information and helpful tips for you.

Please take a few moments to write a review and share it with others on Amazon

Your review might save more lives and help more people.

Thank you, much appreciated!

A SPECIAL GIFT FOR YOU

Unlocks the next secret of

the 21 Days Sugar Detox

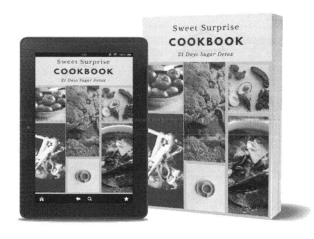

Follow the link below for your detox plan

https://alohatriya.activehosted.com/f/3

ENDNOTES

1. Norris, J. (2009, June 25). Sugar Is a Poison, Says UCSF Obesity Expert. https://www.ucsf.edu/news/2009/06/8187/obesity-and-metabolic-syndrome-driven-fructose-sugar-diet

2. UCSF. (n.d.). The Toxic Truth Too much fructose can damage your liver, just like too much alcohol. Sugar science. https://sugarscience.ucsf.edu/the-toxic-truth/#.YAeYQOlKi9Y

3. 1md organization. (n.d.). How Metabolic Syndrome Occurs and the Role of Sugar in Your Health. https://1md.org/article/how-metabolic-syndrome-occurs-sugar

4. Malik, V. S., Popkin, B. M., Bray, G. A., Després, J. P., Willett, W. C., & Hu, F. B. (2010, Nov.). Sugar-sweetened beverages and risk of metabolic syndrome and type 2 diabetes: 33(11), 2477-2483. https://care.diabetesjournals.org/content/33/11/2477.short

5. Philippou, E. (2018). Are we really what we eat? Nutrition and its role in the onset of rheumatoid arthritis. Autoimmunity Reviews, 17(11), 1074-1077. https://www.sciencedirect.com/science/article/abs/pii/S1568997218302106

6. Touger-Decker, R., & Loveren, C. v. (2003, October). Sugars and dental caries. The American Journal of Clinical Nutrition, 78(4), 881S–892S. https://doi.org/10.1093/ajcn/78.4.881S

7. Gearhardt, A., Yokum, S., Orr, P., Stice, E., Corbin, W., & Brownell, K. (2011). Neural Correlates of Food Addiction. Arch Gen Psychiatry, 68(8), 808–816. doi:10.1001/archgenpsychiatry.2011.32

8. Sack, D. (2013, September 2). 4 Ways Sugar Could Be Harming Your Mental Health. Where Science Meets the Steps. https://www.psychologytoday.com/us/blog/where-science-meets-the-steps/201309/4-ways-sugar-could-be-harming-your-mental-health

9. UCSF. (n.d.). How Much Is Too Much? The growing concern over too much added sugar in our diets. https://sugarscience.ucsf.edu/the-growing-concern-of-overconsumption.html#.YAjuD-lKi9Y

10. WebMD. (2020, October 1). The Truth About Carbs. Carbohydrate's overview. https://www.webmd.com/diet/ss/slideshow-carbohydrates-overview

11. OER Services. (n.d.). Metabolism and Nutrition. Carbohydrate Metabolism. https://courses.lumenlearning.com/suny-ap2/chapter/carbohydrate-metabolism-no-content/

12. What is Starch? - Definition, Function & Chemical Formula. (2016, February 5). https://study.com/academy/lesson/what-is-starch-definition-function-chemical-formula.html

13. Lustig, R. (n.d.). Sugar has 56 Names. https://robertlustig.com/56-names-of-sugar/

14. American diabetes association. (n.d.). Understanding Carbs. Get to Know Carbs. https://www.diabetes.org/healthy-living/recipes-nutrition/understanding-carbs/get-to-know-carbs

15. World public health nutrition association. (2016, January - March). The food system. Food classification, 7(1-3). http://archive.wphna.org/wp-content/uploads/2016/01/WN-2016-7-1-3-28-38-Monteiro-Cannon-Levy-et-al-NOVA.pdf.

16. Whole grains council organization. (n.d.). Gluten free whole grains. whole grain 101. https://wholegrainscouncil.org/whole-grains-101/whats-whole-grain-refined-grain/gluten-free-whole-grains

17. Society for Endocrinology. (n.d.). glands. You and your hormones. https://www.yourhormones.info/glands/

18. Riccardi G, Giacco R, Rivellese AA. Dietary fat, insulin sensitivity and metabolic syndrome. Clin Nutr. 2004 Aug;23(4):447-56. doi: 10.1016/j.clnu.2004.02.006. PMID: 15297079.

19. Nutrition facts organization. (2017, January). What Causes Insulin Resistance? https://nutritionfacts.org/video/What-Causes-Insulin-Resistance/

20. Brown, A. E., & Walker, M. (2016). Genetics of Insulin Resistance and the Metabolic Syndrome. Current cardiology reports, 18(8), 75. https://doi.org/10.1007/s11886-016-0755-4

21. NIDDK. (n.d.). Insulin Resistance & Prediabetes. Diabetes. https://www.niddk.nih.gov/health-information/diabetes/overview/what-is-diabetes/prediabetes-insulin-resistance#insulin

22. National Diabetes Statistics Report, 2020. (2020, August 28). CDC. https://www.cdc.gov/diabetes/data/statistics-report/index.html

23. Diabetes statistics | Professionals. (n.d.). Diabetes UK. Retrieved November 17, 2021, from https://www.diabetes.org.uk/professionals/position-statements-reports/statistics

24. Diagnosis | ADA. (n.d.). American Diabetes Association. https://www.diabetes.org/a1c/diagnosis

25. Basciano H, Federico L, Adeli K. Fructose, insulin resistance, and metabolic dyslipidemia. Nutr Metab (Lond). 2005 Feb 21;2(1):5. doi: 10.1186/1743-7075-2-5. PMID: 15723702; PMCID: PMC552336.

26. Johanna Kuhlmann, Claudia Neumann-Haefelin, Ulrich Belz, Jürgen Kalisch, Hans-Paul Juretschke, Marion Stein, Elke Kleinschmidt, Werner Kramer, Andreas W. Herling

27. Krssak M, Falk Petersen K, Dresner A, DiPietro L, Vogel SM, Rothman DL, Roden M, Shulman GI. Intramyocellular lipid concentrations are correlated with insulin sensitivity in humans: a 1H NMR spectroscopy study. Diabetologia. 1999 Jan;42(1):113-6. doi: 10.1007/s001250051123. Erratum in: Diabetologia 1999 Mar;42(3):386. Erratum in: Diabetologia 1999 Oct;42(10):1269. PMID: 10027589.

28. Nicolaides NC, Chrousos G, Kino T. Glucocorticoid Receptor. [Updated 2020 Nov 21]. In: Feingold KR, Anawalt B, Boyce A, et al., editors. Endotext [Internet]. South Dartmouth (MA): MDText.com, Inc.; 2000-. Available from: https://www.ncbi.nlm.nih.gov/books/NBK279171/

29. Bezdek K and Telzer E (2017) Have No Fear, the Brain is Here! How Your Brain Responds to Stress. Front. Young Minds. 5:71. doi: 10.3389/frym.2017.00071

30. Aloha. (n.d.). Wikipedia. https://en.wikipedia.org/wiki/Aloha

31. Bhattacharya SK, Ghosal S. Anxiolytic activity of a standardized extract of Bacopa monniera: an experimental study. Phytomedicine. 1998 Apr;5(2):77-82. doi: 10.1016/S0944-7113(98)80001-9. PMID: 23195757.

32. Dave UP, Dingankar SR, Saxena VS, Joseph JA, Bethapudi B, Agarwal A, Kudiganti V. An open-label study to elucidate the effects of standardized Bacopa monnieri extract in the management of symptoms of attention-deficit hyperactivity disorder in children. Adv Mind Body Med. 2014 Spring;28(2):10-5. PMID: 24682000.

33. Kamkaew N, Scholfield CN, Ingkaninan K, Maneesai P, Parkington HC, Tare M, Chootip K. Bacopa monnieri and its constituents is hypotensive in anaesthetized rats and vasodilator in various artery types. J Ethnopharmacol. 2011 Sep 1;137(1):790-5. doi: 10.1016/j.jep.2011.06.045. Epub 2011 Jul 5. PMID: 21762768

34. Nemetchek MD, Stierle AA, Stierle DB, Lurie DI. The Ayurvedic plant Bacopa monnieri inhibits inflammatory pathways in the brain. J Ethnopharmacol. 2017 Feb 2;197:92-100. doi: 10.1016/j.jep.2016.07.073. Epub 2016 Jul 26. PMID: 27473605; PMCID: PMC5269610.

35. Smith E, Palethorpe HM, Tomita Y, Pei JV, Townsend AR, Price TJ, Young JP, Yool AJ, Hardingham JE. The Purified Extract from the Medicinal Plant Bacopa monnieri, Bacopaside II, Inhibits Growth of Colon Cancer Cells In Vitro by Inducing Cell Cycle Arrest and Apoptosis. Cells. 2018 Jul 21;7(7):81. doi: 10.3390/cells7070081. PMID: 30037060; PMCID: PMC6070819.

36. Vollala VR, Upadhya S, Nayak S. Enhancement of basolateral amygdaloid neuronal dendritic arborization following Bacopa monniera extract treatment in adult rats. Clinics (Sao Paulo). 2011;66(4):663-71. doi: 10.1590/s1807-59322011000400023. PMID: 21655763; PMCID: PMC3093798.

37. Marshall-Pescini, S., Schaebs, F. S., Gaugg, A., Meinert, A., Deschner, T., & Range, F. (2019). The Role of Oxytocin in the Dog-Owner Relationship. Animals : an open access journal from MDPI, 9(10), 792. https://doi.org/10.3390/ani9100792

38. DiNicolantonio, J., O'Keefe, J., & Wilson, W. (2018). Sugar addiction: is it real? A narrative review British Journal of Sports Medicine, (52), 910-913. https://bjsm.bmj.com/content/52/14/910

39. Murray, K. (2020, November 20). Sugar Addiction. https://www.addictioncenter.com/drugs/sugar-addiction/

40. Hormone Health Network."Serotonin | Hormone Health Network." Hormone.org, Endocrine Society, 3 February 2021, https://www.hormone.org/your-health-and-hormones/glands-and-hormones-a-to-z/hormones/serotonin

41. Kent, J. (2020, April 12). Real Reason #5 for Sugar Cravings: Serotonin. https://medium.com/illumination/real-reason-5-for-sugar-cravings-serotonin-c4b55105396a

42. Whitbread, D. (n.d.). MyFoodData Foods Lists. MyFoodData Foods Lists. https://www.myfooddata.com/articles/

43. Wipfli, B., Landers, D., Nagoshi, C. and Ringenbach, S. (2011), An examination of serotonin and psychological variables in the relationship between exercise and mental health. Scandinavian Journal of Medicine & Science in Sports, 21: 474-481. https://doi.org/10.1111/j.1600-0838.2009.01049.x

44. Lambert GW, Reid C, Kaye DM, Jennings GL, Esler MD. Effect of sunlight and season on serotonin turnover in the brain. Lancet. 2002 Dec 7;360(9348):1840-2. doi: 10.1016/s0140-6736(02)11737-5. PMID: 12480364.

45. Nathaniel Mead, M. (2008, April 1). Benefits of Sunlight: A Bright Spot for Human Health. Environews, 116(4). https://doi.org/10.1289/ehp.116-a160

46. Krishnakumar, D., Hamblin, M. R., & Lakshmanan, S. (2015). Meditation and Yoga can Modulate Brain Mechanisms that affect Behavior and Anxiety-A Modern Scientific Perspective. Ancient science, 2(1), 13–19. https://doi.org/10.14259/as.v2i1.171

47. Athilingam, J. C., Ben-Shalom, R., Keeshen, C. M., Sohal, V. S., & Bender, K. J. (2017). Serotonin enhances excitability and gamma frequency temporal integration in mouse prefrontal fast-spiking interneurons. eLife, 6, e31991. https://doi.org/10.7554/eLife.31991

48. Heijnen, S., Hommel, B., Kibele, A., & Colzato, L. S. (2016). Neuromodulation of Aerobic Exercise-A Review. Frontiers in psychology, 6, 1890. https://doi.org/10.3389/fpsyg.2015.01890

49. Jun Pang, Zheng Zhang, Tong-zhang Zheng, Bryan A. Bassig, Chen Mao, Xingbin Liu, Yong Zhu, Kunchong Shi, Junbo Ge, Yue-jin Yang, Dejia-Huang, Ming Bai, Yu Peng,

50. Mandal, Ananya. (2019, April 09). Dopamine Functions. News-Medical. Retrieved on February 06, 2021, from https://www.news-medical.net/health/Dopamine-Functions.aspx.

51. Vilímovský, M. (2014, December 18). Low dopamine (e.g., dopamine deficiency): causes, symptoms, diagnosis and treatment options. Health A-Z.

52. Whitbread, D. (n.d.). MyFoodData Foods Lists. MyFoodData Foods Lists. https://www.myfooddata.com/articles/

53. Sutoo D, Akiyama K. Regulation of brain function by exercise. Neurobiol Dis. 2003 Jun;13(1):1-14. doi: 10.1016/s0969-9961(03)00030-5. PMID: 12758062.

54. Erkkilä J, Punkanen M, Fachner J, Ala-Ruona E, Pöntiö I, Tervaniemi M, Vanhala M, Gold C. Individual music therapy for depression: randomised controlled trial. Br J Psychiatry. 2011 Aug;199(2):132-9. doi: 10.1192/bjp.bp.110.085431. Epub 2011 Apr 7. PMID: 21474494.

55. Salimpoor, V., Benovoy, M., Larcher, K. et al. Anatomically distinct dopamine release during anticipation and experience of peak emotion to music. Nat Neurosci 14, 257–262 (2011). https://doi.org/10.1038/nn.2726

56. Harvard medical school. (2011, April). In the journals: Mindfulness meditation practice changes the brain. Harvard Women's Health Watch. https://www.health.harvard.edu/mind-and-mood/mindfulness-meditation-practice-changes-the-brain

57. Xie L, Kang H, Xu Q, Chen MJ, Liao Y, Thiyagarajan M, O'Donnell J, Christensen DJ, Nicholson C, Iliff JJ, Takano T, Deane R, Nedergaard M. Sleep drives metabolite clearance from the adult brain. Science. 2013 Oct 18;342(6156):373-7. doi: 10.1126/science.1241224. PMID: 24136970; PMCID: PMC3880190.

58. Field T, Hernandez-Reif M, Diego M, Schanberg S, Kuhn C. Cortisol decreases, and serotonin and dopamine increase following massage therapy. Int J Neurosci. 2005 Oct;115(10):1397-413. doi: 10.1080/00207450590956459. PMID: 16162447.

59. National Center for Biotechnology Information (2021). PubChem Compound Summary for CID 34756, S-Adenosyl-L-methionine. Retrieved February 15, 2021, from https://pubchem.ncbi.nlm.nih.gov/compound/S-Adenosyl-L-methionine.

60. Jun Pang, Zheng Zhang, Tong-zhang Zheng, Bryan A. Bassig, Chen Mao, Xingbin Liu, Yong Zhu, Kunchong Shi, Junbo Ge, Yue-jin Yang, Dejia-Huang, Ming Bai, Yu Peng,

61. Nathan PJ, Lu K, Gray M, Oliver C. The neuropharmacology of L-theanine(N-ethyl-L-glutamine): a possible neuroprotective and cognitive enhancing agent. J Herb Pharmacother. 2006;6(2):21-30. PMID: 17182482.

62. Lampariello, L. R., Cortelazzo, A., Guerranti, R., Sticozzi, C., & Valacchi, G. (2012). The Magic Velvet Bean of Mucuna pruriens. Journal of traditional and complementary medicine, 2(4), 331–339. https://doi.org/10.1016/s2225-4110(16)30119-5

63. Jezova D, Duncko R, Lassanova M, Kriska M, Moncek F. Reduction of rise in blood pressure and cortisol release during stress by Ginkgo biloba extract (EGb 761) in healthy volunteers. J Physiol Pharmacol. 2002 Sep;53(3):337-48. PMID: 12369732

64. Ramassamy C, Naudin B, Christen Y, Clostre F, Costentin J. Prevention by Ginkgo biloba extract (EGb 761) and trolox C of the decrease in synaptosomal dopamine or serotonin uptake following incubation. Biochem Pharmacol. 1992 Dec 15;44(12):2395-401. doi: 10.1016/0006-2952(92)90685-c. PMID: 1472105.

65. Thomas RB, Joy S, Ajayan MS, Paulose CS. Neuroprotective potential of Bacopa monnieri and Bacoside A against dopamine receptor dysfunction in the cerebral cortex of neonatal hypoglycaemia rats. Cell Mol Neurobiol. 2013 Nov;33(8):1065-74. doi: 10.1007/s10571-013-9973-0. Epub 2013 Aug 22. PMID: 23975094.

66. Bode AM, Dong Z. The Amazing and Mighty Ginger. In: Benzie IFF, Wachtel-Galor S, editors. Herbal Medicine: Biomolecular and Clinical Aspects. 2nd edition. Boca Raton (FL): CRC Press/Taylor & Francis; 2011. Chapter 7. Available from: https://www.ncbi.nlm.nih.gov/books/NBK92775/

67. Mashhadi, N. S., Ghiasvand, R., Askari, G., Hariri, M., Darvishi, L., & Mofid, M. R. (2013). Anti-oxidative and anti-inflammatory effects of ginger in health and physical activity: review of current evidence. International journal of preventive medicine, 4(Suppl 1), S36–S42.

68. Masuda Y, Kikuzaki H, Hisamoto M, Nakatani N. Antioxidant properties of gingerol related compounds from ginger. Biofactors. 2004;21(1-4):293-6. doi: 10.1002/biof.552210157. PMID: 15630214.

69. HyunKim, K., Lee, D., Lee, L., Kim, C.-E., Jung, K. w., & Kang, S. (2018, July). Beneficial effects of Panax ginseng for the treatment and prevention of neurodegenerative diseases: past findings and future directions. Journal of Ginseng Research, 42(3), 239-247. https://doi.org/10.1016/j.jgr.2017.03.011

70. Kim CS, Park JB, Kim KJ, Chang SJ, Ryoo SW, Jeon BH. Effect of Korea red ginseng on cerebral blood flow and superoxide production. Acta Pharmacol Sin. 2002 Dec;23(12):1152-6. PMID: 12466053.

71. Lee, S. H., Park, W. S., & Lim, M. H. (2011). Clinical effects of korean red ginseng on attention deficit hyperactivity disorder in children: an observational study. Journal of ginseng research, 35(2), 226–234. https://doi.org/10.5142/jgr.2011.35.2.226

72. Kevin Yue Zhu, Qing-Qiu Mao, Siu-Po Ip, Roy Chi-Yan Choi, Tina Ting-Xia Dong, David Tai-Wai Lau, Karl Wah-Keung Tsim, "A Standardized Chinese Herbal Decoction, Kai-Xin-San, Restores Decreased Levels of Neurotransmitters and Neurotrophic Factors in the Brain of Chronic Stress-Induced Depressive Rats", Evidence-Based Complementary and Alternative Medicine, vol. 2012, Article ID 149256, 13 pages, 2012. https://doi.org/10.1155/2012/149256

73. Kulkarni, S.K., Bhutani, M.K. & Bishnoi, M. Antidepressant activity of curcumin: involvement of serotonin and dopamine system. Psychopharmacology 201, 435 (2008). https://doi.org/10.1007/s00213-008-1300-y

74. Bhat A, Mahalakshmi AM, Ray B, Tuladhar S, Hediyal TA, Manthiannem E, Padamati J, Chandra R, Chidambaram SB, Sakharkar MK. Benefits of curcumin in brain disorders. Biofactors. 2019 Sep;45(5):666-689. doi: 10.1002/biof.1533. Epub 2019 Jun 11. PMID: 31185140.

75. Breit, S., Kupferberg, A., Rogler, G., & Hasler, G. (2018). Vagus Nerve as Modulator of the Brain-Gut Axis in Psychiatric and Inflammatory Disorders. Frontiers in psychiatry, 9, 44. https://doi.org/10.3389/fpsyt.2018.00044

76. Yano, J. M., Yu, K., Donaldson, G. P., Shastri, G. G., Ann, P., Ma, L., Nagler, C. R., Ismagilov, R. F., Mazmanian, S. K., & Hsiao, E. Y. (2015). Indigenous bacteria from the gut microbiota regulate host serotonin biosynthesis. Cell, 161(2), 264–276. https://doi.org/10.1016/j.cell.2015.02.047

77. Xue, R., Zhang, H., Pan, J., Du, Z., Zhou, W., Zhang, Z., Tian, Z., Zhou, R., & Bai, L. (2018). Peripheral Dopamine Controlled by Gut Microbes Inhibits Invariant Natural Killer T Cell-Mediated Hepatitis. Frontiers in immunology, 9, 2398. https://doi.org/10.3389/fimmu.2018.02398

78. Thursby, E., & Juge, N. (2017). Introduction to the human gut microbiota. The Biochemical journal, 474(11), 1823–1836. https://doi.org/10.1042/BCJ20160510

79. Quigley E. M. (2013). Gut bacteria in health and disease. Gastroenterology & hepatology, 9(9), 560–569.

80. Hernández, M., Canfora, E. E., Jocken, J., & Blaak, E. E. (2019). Short-Chain Fatty Acid Acetate in Body Weight Control and Insulin Sensitivity. Nutrients, 11(8), 1943. https://doi.org/10.3390/nu11081943

81. Bourassa, M. W., Alim, I., Bultman, S. J., & Ratan, R. R. (2016). Butyrate, neuroepigenetics and the gut microbiome: Can a high fiber diet improve brain health? Neuroscience letters, 625, 56–63. https://doi.org/10.1016/j.neulet.2016.02.009

82. Li, Q., Cao, L., Tian, Y., Zhang, P., Ding, C., Lu, W., Jia, C., Shao, C., Liu, W., Wang, D., Ye, H., & Hao, H. (2018). Butyrate Suppresses the Proliferation of Colorectal Cancer Cells via Targeting Pyruvate Kinase M2 and Metabolic Reprogramming. Molecular & cellular proteomics : MCP, 17(8), 1531–1545. https://doi.org/10.1074/mcp.RA118.000752

83. McNabney, S. M., & Henagan, T. M. (2017). Short Chain Fatty Acids in the Colon and Peripheral Tissues: A Focus on Butyrate, Colon Cancer, Obesity and Insulin Resistance. Nutrients, 9(12), 1348. https://doi.org/10.3390/nu9121348

84. Li, Z., Yi, C. X., Katiraei, S., Kooijman, S., Zhou, E., Chung, C. K., Gao, Y., van den Heuvel, J. K., Meijer, O. C., Berbée, J., Heijink, M., Giera, M., Willems van Dijk, K., Groen, A. K., Rensen, P., & Wang, Y. (2018). Butyrate reduces appetite and activates brown adipose tissue via the gut-brain neural circuit. Gut, 67(7), 1269–1279. https://doi.org/10.1136/gutjnl-2017-314050

85. Hou, Y. F., Shan, C., Zhuang, S. Y., Zhuang, Q. Q., Ghosh, A., Zhu, K. C., Kong, X. K., Wang, S. M., Gong, Y. L., Yang, Y. Y., Tao, B., Sun, L. H., Zhao, H. Y., Guo, X. Z., Wang, W. Q., Ning, G., Gu, Y. Y., Li, S. T., & Liu, J. M. (2021). Gut microbiota-derived propionate mediates the neuroprotective effect of osteocalcin in a mouse model of Parkinson's disease. Microbiome, 9(1), 34. https://doi.org/10.1186/s40168-020-00988-6

86. Kim, K., Kwon, O., Ryu, T. Y., Jung, C. R., Kim, J., Min, J. K., Kim, D. S., Son, M. Y., & Cho, H. S. (2019). Propionate of a microbiota metabolite induces cell apoptosis and cell cycle arrest in lung cancer. Molecular medicine reports, 20(2), 1569–1574. https://doi.org/10.3892/mmr.2019.10431

87. van Limpt, C., Crienen, A., Vriesema, A. et al. 134 Effect of Colonic Short Chain Fatty Acids, Lactate and PH on The Growth of Common Gut Pathogens. Pediatr Res 56, 487 (2004). https://doi.org/10.1203/00006450-200409000-00157

88. Colombo, M., Castilho, N.P.A., Todorov, S.D. et al. Beneficial properties of lactic acid bacteria naturally present in dairy production. BMC Microbiol 18, 219 (2018). https://doi.org/10.1186/s12866-018-1356-8

89. King, S., Glanville, J., Sanders, M. E., Fitzgerald, A., & Varley, D. (2014). Effectiveness of probiotics on the duration of illness in healthy children and adults who develop common acute respiratory infectious conditions: a systematic review and meta-analysis. The British journal of nutrition, 112(1), 41–54. https://doi.org/10.1017/S0007114514000075

90. Leyer, G. J., Li, S., Mubasher, M. E., Reifer, C., & Ouwehand, A. C. (2009). Probiotic effects on cold and influenza-like symptom incidence and duration in children. Pediatrics, 124(2), e172–e179. https://doi.org/10.1542/peds.2008-2666

91. Leyer, G. J., Li, S., Mubasher, M. E., Reifer, C., & Ouwehand, A. C. (2009). Probiotic effects on cold and influenza-like symptom incidence and duration in children. Pediatrics, 124(2), e172–e179. https://doi.org/10.1542/peds.2008-2666

92. Riske, L., Thomas, R. K., Baker, G. B., & Dursun, S. M. (2017). Lactate in the brain: an update on its relevance to brain energy, neurons, glia and panic disorder. Therapeutic advances in psychopharmacology, 7(2), 85–89. https://doi.org/10.1177/2045125316675579

93. Caspani, G., Kennedy, S., Foster, J. A., & Swann, J. (2019). Gut microbial metabolites in depression: understanding the biochemical mechanisms. Microbial cell (Graz, Austria), 6(10), 454–481. https://doi.org/10.15698/mic2019.10.693

94. Thursby, E., & Juge, N. (2017). Introduction to the human gut microbiota. The Biochemical journal, 474(11), 1823–1836. https://doi.org/10.1042/BCJ20160510

95. Fang, H., Kang, J., & Zhang, D. (2017). Microbial production of vitamin B12: a review and future perspectives. Microbial cell factories, 16(1), 15. https://doi.org/10.1186/s12934-017-0631-y

96. LeBlanc, J., Laiño, J., del Valle, M.J., Vannini, V., van Sinderen, D., Taranto, M., de Valdez, G.F., de Giori, G.S. and Sesma, F. (2011), B-Group vitamin production by lactic acid bacteria – current knowledge and potential applications. Journal of Applied Microbiology, 111: 1297-1309. https://doi.org/10.1111/j.1365-2672.2011.05157.x

97. Elizabeth Thursby, Nathalie Juge; Introduction to the human gut microbiota. Biochem J 1 June 2017; 474 (11): 1823–1836. doi: https://doi.org/10.1042/BCJ20160510

98. Patel, R. M., & Denning, P. W. (2013). Therapeutic use of prebiotics, probiotics, and postbiotics to prevent necrotizing enterocolitis: what is the current evidence? Clinics in perinatology, 40(1), 11–25. https://doi.org/10.1016/j.clp.2012.12.002

99. Myhrstad, M., Tunsjø, H., Charnock, C., & Telle-Hansen, V. H. (2020). Dietary Fiber, Gut Microbiota, and Metabolic Regulation-Current Status in Human Randomized Trials. Nutrients, 12(3), 859. https://doi.org/10.3390/nu12030859

100. van de Wiele, T., Boon, N., Possemiers, S., Jacobs, H., & Verstraete, W. (2007). Inulin-type fructans of longer degree of polymerization exert more pronounced in vitro prebiotic effects. Journal of applied microbiology, 102(2), 452–460. https://doi.org/10.1111/j.1365-2672.2006.03084.x

101. Carlson, J. L., Erickson, J. M., Lloyd, B. B., & Slavin, J. L. (2018). Health Effects and Sources of Prebiotic Dietary Fiber. Current developments in nutrition, 2(3), nzy005. https://doi.org/10.1093/cdn/nzy005

102. Boyer, J., & Liu, R. H. (2004). Apple phytochemicals and their health benefits. Nutrition journal, 3, 5. https://doi.org/10.1186/1475-2891-3-5

103. Mohamed A. Awad, Anton de Jager, Lucie M. van Westing,Flavonoid and chlorogenic acid levels in apple fruit: characterisation of variation,Scientia Horticulturae,Volume 83, Issues 3–4,2000,Pages 249-263,ISSN 0304-4238,https://doi.org/10.1016/S0304-4238(99)00124-7.

104. Licht, T. R., Hansen, M., Bergström, A., Poulsen, M., Krath, B. N., Markowski, J., Dragsted, L. O., & Wilcks, A. (2010). Effects of apples and specific apple components on the cecal environment of conventional rats: role of apple pectin. BMC microbiology, 10, 13. https://doi.org/10.1186/1471-2180-10-13

105. Jiang, T., Gao, X., Wu, C., Tian, F., Lei, Q., Bi, J., Xie, B., Wang, H. Y., Chen, S., & Wang, X. (2016). Apple-Derived Pectin Modulates Gut Microbiota, Improves Gut Barrier Function, and Attenuates Metabolic Endotoxemia in Rats with Diet-Induced Obesity. Nutrients, 8(3), 126. https://doi.org/10.3390/nu8030126

106. Koutsos, A., Tuohy, K. M., & Lovegrove, J. A. (2015). Apples and cardiovascular health--is the gut microbiota a core consideration? Nutrients, 7(6), 3959–3998. https://doi.org/10.3390/nu7063959

107. Slavin J. (2013). Fiber and prebiotics: mechanisms and health benefits. Nutrients, 5(4), 1417–1435. https://doi.org/10.3390/nu5041417

108. Snelson, M., Jong, J., Manolas, D., Kok, S., Louise, A., Stern, R., & Kellow, N. J. (2019). Metabolic Effects of Resistant Starch Type 2: A Systematic Literature Review and Meta-Analysis of Randomized Controlled Trials. Nutrients, 11(8), 1833. https://doi.org/10.3390/nu11081833

109. Thaísa Menezes Alves Moro, Caroline Mantovani Celegatti, Ana Paula Aparecida Pereira, Aline Sousa Lopes, Douglas Fernandes Barbin, Glaucia Maria Pastore, Maria Teresa Pedrosa Silva Clerici,Use of burdock root flour as a prebiotic ingredient in cookies,LWT,Volume 90,2018,Pages 540-546,ISSN 0023-6430. https://doi.org/10.1016/j.lwt.2017.12.059.

110. Sorrenti, V., Ali, S., Mancin, L., Davinelli, S., Paoli, A., & Scapagnini, G. (2020). Cocoa Polyphenols and Gut Microbiota Interplay: Bioavailability, Prebiotic Effect, and Impact on Human Health. Nutrients, 12(7), 1908. https://doi.org/10.3390/nu12071908

111. Nishimura, M., Ohkawara, T., Kanayama, T., Kitagawa, K., Nishimura, H., & Nishihira, J. (2015). Effects of the extract from roasted chicory (Cichorium intybus L.) root containing inulin-type fructans on blood glucose, lipid metabolism, and fecal properties. Journal of traditional and complementary medicine, 5(3), 161–167. https://doi.org/10.1016/j.jtcme.2014.11.016

112. Wirngo, F. E., Lambert, M. N., & Jeppesen, P. B. (2016). The Physiological Effects of Dandelion (Taraxacum Officinale) in Type 2 Diabetes. The review of diabetic studies : RDS, 13(2-3), 113–131. https://doi.org/10.1900/RDS.2016.13.113

113. Bernadetta Lis, Beata Olas,Pro-health activity of dandelion (Taraxacum officinale L.) and its food products – history and present,Journal of Functional Foods,Volume 59,2019,Pages 40-48,ISSN 1756-4646,https://doi.org/10.1016/j.jff.2019.05.012.

114. Thumann, T. A., Pferschy-Wenzig, E. M., Moissl-Eichinger, C., & Bauer, R. (2019). The role of gut microbiota for the activity of medicinal plants traditionally used in the European Union for gastrointestinal disorders. Journal of ethnopharmacology, 245, 112153. https://doi.org/10.1016/j.jep.2019.112153

115. Kajla, P., Sharma, A., & Sood, D. R. (2015). Flaxseed-a potential functional food source. Journal of food science and technology, 52(4), 1857–1871. https://doi.org/10.1007/s13197-014-1293-y

116. Chen, K., Nakasone, Y., Xie, K., Sakao, K., & Hou, D. X. (2020). Modulation of Allicin-Free Garlic on Gut Microbiome. Molecules (Basel, Switzerland), 25(3), 682. https://doi.org/10.3390/molecules25030682

117. Ning Zhang, Xuesong Huang, Yanhua Zeng, Xiyang Wu, Xichun Peng,Study on prebiotic effectiveness of neutral garlic fructan in vitro,Food Science and Human Wellness,Volume 2, Issues 3–4,2013,Pages 119-123,ISSN 2213-4530,https://doi.org/10.1016/j.fshw.2013.07.001.

118. Behera, S. S., & Ray, R. C. (2016). Konjac glucomannan, a promising polysaccharide of Amorphophallus konjac K. Koch in health care. International Journal of biological macromolecules, 92, 942–956. https://doi.org/10.1016/j.ijbiomac.2016.07.098

119. Yin, J. Y., Ma, L. Y., Xie, M. Y., Nie, S. P., & Wu, J. Y. (2020). Molecular properties and gut health benefits of enzyme-hydrolyzed konjac glucomannans. Carbohydrate polymers, 237, 116117. https://doi.org/10.1016/j.carbpol.2020.116117

120. Tester, R. F., & Al-Ghazzewi, F. H. (2016). Beneficial health characteristics of native and hydrolysed konjac (Amorphophallus konjac) glucomannan. Journal of the science of food and agriculture, 96(10), 3283–3291. https://doi.org/10.1002/jsfa.7571

121. Sawicka, B., Skiba, D., Pszczółkowski, P., Aslan, I., Sharifi-Rad, J., & Krochmal-Marczak, B. (2020). Jerusalem artichoke (Helianthus tuberosus L.) as a medicinal plant and its natural products. Cellular and molecular biology (Noisy-le-Grand, France), 66(4), 160–177.

122. Park, C. J., & Han, J. S. (2015). Hypoglycemic Effect of Jicama (Pachyrhizus erosus) Extract on Streptozotocin-Induced Diabetic Mice. Preventive nutrition and food science, 20(2), 88–93. https://doi.org/10.3746/pnf.2015.20.2.88

123. Escobar-Ledesma, F. R., Sánchez-Moreno, V. E., Vera, E., Ciobotă, V., Jentzsch, P. V., & Jaramillo, L. I. (2020). Extraction of Inulin from Andean Plants: An Approach to Non-Traditional Crops of Ecuador. Molecules (Basel, Switzerland), 25(21), 5067. https://doi.org/10.3390/molecules25215067

124. Kumar, V. P., Prashanth, K., & Venkatesh, Y. P. (2015). Structural analyses and immunomodulatory properties of fructo-oligosaccharides from onion (Allium cepa). Carbohydrate polymers, 117, 115–122. https://doi.org/10.1016/j.carbpol.2014.09.039

125. Justin L Carlson, Jennifer M Erickson, Beate B Lloyd, Joanne L Slavin, Health Effects and Sources of Prebiotic Dietary Fiber, Current Developments in Nutrition, Volume 2, Issue 3, March 2018, nzy005, https://doi.org/10.1093/cdn/nzy005

126. Nicastro, H. L., Ross, S. A., & Milner, J. A. (2015). Garlic and onions: their cancer prevention properties. Cancer prevention research (Philadelphia, Pa.), 8(3), 181–189. https://doi.org/10.1158/1940-6207.CAPR-14-0172

127. Mlcek, J., Jurikova, T., Skrovankova, S., & Sochor, J. (2016). Quercetin and Its Anti-Allergic Immune Response. Molecules (Basel, Switzerland), 21(5), 623. https://doi.org/10.3390/molecules21050623

128. Suleria, H. A., Butt, M. S., Anjum, F. M., Saeed, F., & Khalid, N. (2015). Onion: nature protection against physiological threats. Critical reviews in food science and nutrition, 55(1), 50–66. https://doi.org/10.1080/10408398.2011.646364

129. Peñalver, R., Lorenzo, J. M., Ros, G., Amarowicz, R., Pateiro, M., & Nieto, G. (2020). Seaweeds as a Functional Ingredient for a Healthy Diet. Marine drugs, 18(6), 301. https://doi.org/10.3390/md18060301

130. Chen, L., Xu, W., Chen, D., Chen, G., Liu, J., Zeng, X., Shao, R., & Zhu, H. (2018). Digestibility of sulfated polysaccharide from the brown seaweed Ascophyllum nodosum and its effect on the human gut microbiota in vitro. International journal of biological macromolecules, 112, 1055–1061. https://doi.org/10.1016/j.ijbiomac.2018.01.183

131. Maki, K. C., Gibson, G. R., Dickmann, R. S., Kendall, C. W., Chen, C. Y., Costabile, A., Comelli, E. M., McKay, D. L., Almeida, N. G., Jenkins, D., Zello, G. A., & Blumberg, J. B. (2012). Digestive and physiologic effects of a wheat bran extract, arabino-xylan-oligosaccharide, in breakfast cereal. Nutrition (Burbank, Los Angeles County, Calif.), 28(11-12), 1115–1121. https://doi.org/10.1016/j.nut.2012.02.010

132. Cloetens, L., Broekaert, W. F., Delaedt, Y., Ollevier, F., Courtin, C. M., Delcour, J. A., Rutgeerts, P., & Verbeke, K. (2010). Tolerance of arabinoxylan-oligosaccharides and their prebiotic activity in healthy subjects: a randomised, placebo-controlled cross-over study. The British journal of nutrition, 103(5), 703–713. https://doi.org/10.1017/S0007114509992248

133. François, I. E., Lescroart, O., Veraverbeke, W. S., Marzorati, M., Possemiers, S., Hamer, H., Windey, K., Welling, G. W., Delcour, J. A., Courtin, C. M., Verbeke, K., & Broekaert, W. F. (2014). Effects of wheat bran extract containing arabinoxylan oligosaccharides on gastrointestinal parameters in healthy preadolescent children. Journal of pediatric gastroenterology and nutrition, 58(5), 647–653. https://doi.org/10.1097/MPG.0000000000000285

134. Jefferson, A., & Adolphus, K. (2019). The Effects of Intact Cereal Grain Fibers, Including Wheat Bran on the Gut Microbiota Composition of Healthy Adults: A Systematic Review. Frontiers in nutrition, 6, 33. https://doi.org/10.3389/fnut.2019.00033

135. Damen, B., Cloetens, L., Broekaert, W. F., François, I., Lescroart, O., Trogh, I., Arnaut, F., Welling, G. W., Wijffels, J., Delcour, J. A., Verbeke, K., & Courtin, C. M. (2012). Consumption of breads containing in situ-produced arabinoxylan oligosaccharides alters gastrointestinal effects in healthy volunteers. The Journal of nutrition, 142(3), 470–477. https://doi.org/10.3945/jn.111.146464

136. Kjølbæk, L., Benítez-Páez, A., Gómez Del Pulgar, E. M., Brahe, L. K., Liebisch, G., Matysik, S., Rampelli, S., Vermeiren, J., Brigidi, P., Larsen, L. H., Astrup, A., & Sanz, Y. (2020). Arabinoxylan oligosaccharides and polyunsaturated fatty acid effects on

gut microbiota and metabolic markers in overweight individuals with signs of metabolic syndrome: A randomized cross-over trial. Clinical nutrition (Edinburgh, Scotland), 39(1), 67–79. https://doi.org/10.1016/j.clnu.2019.01.012

137. Caetano, B. F., de Moura, N. A., Almeida, A. P., Dias, M. C., Sivieri, K., & Barbisan, L. F. (2016). Yacon (Smallanthus sonchifolius) as a Food Supplement: Health-Promoting Benefits of Fructooligosaccharides. Nutrients, 8(7), 436. https://doi.org/10.3390/nu8070436

138. Delgado, G. T., Tamashiro, W. M., Maróstica Junior, M. R., & Pastore, G. M. (2013). Yacon (Smallanthus sonchifolius): a functional food. Plant foods for human nutrition (Dordrecht, Netherlands), 68(3), 222–228. https://doi.org/10.1007/s11130-013-0362-0

139. Birt, D. F., Boylston, T., Hendrich, S., Jane, J. L., Hollis, J., Li, L., McClelland, J., Moore, S., Phillips, G. J., Rowling, M., Schalinske, K., Scott, M. P., & Whitley, E. M. (2013). Resistant starch: promise for improving human health. Advances in nutrition (Bethesda, Md.), 4(6), 587–601. https://doi.org/10.3945/an.113.004325

140. Topping, D. L., & Clifton, P. M. (2001). Short-chain fatty acids and human colonic function: roles of resistant starch and nonstarch polysaccharides. Physiological reviews, 81(3), 1031–1064. https://doi.org/10.1152/physrev.2001.81.3.1031

141. Arena, M. P., Caggianiello, G., Fiocco, D., Russo, P., Torelli, M., Spano, G., & Capozzi, V. (2014). Barley β-glucans-containing food enhances probiotic performances of beneficial bacteria. International journal of molecular sciences, 15(2), 3025–3039. https://doi.org/10.3390/ijms15023025

142. D. El Khoury, C. Cuda, B. L. Luhovyy, G. H. Anderson, "Beta Glucan: Health Benefits in Obesity and Metabolic Syndrome", Journal of Nutrition and Metabolism, vol. 2012, Article ID 851362, 28 pages, 2012. https://doi.org/10.1155/2012/851362

143. Shen, X. L., Zhao, T., Zhou, Y., Shi, X., Zou, Y., & Zhao, G. (2016). Effect of Oat β-Glucan Intake on Glycaemic Control and Insulin Sensitivity of Diabetic Patients: A Meta-Analysis of Randomized Controlled Trials. Nutrients, 8(1), 39. https://doi.org/10.3390/nu8010039

144. Valeur, J., Puaschitz, N. G., Midtvedt, T., & Berstad, A. (2016). Oatmeal porridge: impact on microflora-associated characteristics in healthy subjects. The British journal of nutrition, 115(1), 62–67. https://doi.org/10.1017/S0007114515004213

145. Aryana, K. J., & Olson, D. W. (2017). A 100-Year Review: Yogurt and other cultured dairy products. Journal of dairy science, 100(12), 9987–10013. https://doi.org/10.3168/jds.2017-12981

146. J.M. Kongo, F.X. Malcata,Acidophilus Milk,Editor(s): Benjamin Caballero, Paul M. Finglas, Fidel Toldrá,

147. Gilliland S. E. (1989). Acidophilus milk products: a review of potential benefits to consumers. Journal of dairy science, 72(10), 2483–2494. https://doi.org/10.3168/jds.S0022-0302(89)79389-9

148. de Oliveira Leite, A. M., Miguel, M. A., Peixoto, R. S., Rosado, A. S., Silva, J. T., & Paschoalin, V. M. (2013). Microbiological, technological and therapeutic properties of kefir: a natural probiotic beverage. Brazilian journal of microbiology : [publication of the Brazilian Society for Microbiology], 44(2), 341–349. https://doi.org/10.1590/S1517-83822013000200001

149. Bourrie, B. C., Willing, B. P., & Cotter, P. D. (2016). The Microbiota and Health Promoting Characteristics of the Fermented Beverage Kefir. Frontiers in microbiology, 7, 647. https://doi.org/10.3389/fmicb.2016.00647

150. Park, K. Y., Jeong, J. K., Lee, Y. E., & Daily, J. W., 3rd (2014). Health benefits of kimchi (Korean fermented vegetables) as a probiotic food. Journal of medicinal food, 17(1), 6–20. https://doi.org/10.1089/jmf.2013.3083

151. Patra, J. K., Das, G., Paramithiotis, S., & Shin, H. S. (2016). Kimchi and Other Widely Consumed Traditional Fermented Foods of Korea: A Review. Frontiers in microbiology, 7, 1493. https://doi.org/10.3389/fmicb.2016.01493

152. Jayabalan, R., Malbaša, R.V., Lončar, E.S., Vitas, J.S. and Sathishkumar, M. (2014), A Review on Kombucha Tea—Microbiology, Composition, Fermentation, Beneficial Effects, Toxicity, and Tea Fungus. Comprehensive Reviews in Food Science and Food Safety, 13: 538-550. https://doi.org/10.1111/1541-4337.12073

153. Villarreal-Soto, S. A., Beaufort, S., Bouajila, J., Souchard, J. P., & Taillandier, P. (2018). Understanding Kombucha Tea Fermentation: A Review. Journal of food science, 83(3), 580–588. https://doi.org/10.1111/1750-3841.14068

154. wikipedia organization. (2021, June 23). Kumis. https://en.wikipedia.org/wiki/Kumis

155. Tang, H., Ma, H., Hou, Q., Li, W., Xu, H., Liu, W., Sun, Z., Haobisi, H., & Menghe, B. (2020). Profiling of koumiss microbiota and organic acids and their effects on koumiss taste. BMC microbiology, 20(1), 85. https://doi.org/10.1186/s12866-020-01773-z

156. Behera, Dr. Sunil & Panda, Sandeep & Kayitesi, Eugenie & Mulaba-Bafubiandi, Antoine. (2017). Kefir and Koumiss Origin, Health Benefits and Current Status of Knowledge. https://www.researchgate.net/publication/316824128_Kefir_and_Koumiss_Origin_Health_Benefits_and_Current_Status_of_Knowledge

157. Abdel-Salam, A. M., Al-Dekheil, A., Babkr, A., Farahna, M., & Mousa, H. M. (2010). High fiber probiotic fermented mare's milk reduces the toxic effects of mercury in rats. North American journal of medical sciences, 2(12), 569–575. https://doi.org/10.4297/najms.2010.2569

158. Riaz Rajoka, M. S., Mehwish, H. M., Zhang, H., Ashraf, M., Fang, H., Zeng, X., Wu, Y., Khurshid, M., Zhao, L., & He, Z. (2020). Antibacterial and antioxidant activity of exopolysaccharide mediated silver nanoparticle synthesized by Lactobacillus brevis isolated from Chinese koumiss. Colloids and surfaces. B, Biointerfaces, 186, 110734. https://doi.org/10.1016/j.colsurfb.2019.110734

159. Yerlikaya, OktayStarter cultures used in probiotic dairy product preparation and popular probiotic dairy drinks. Food Science and Technology [online]. 2014, v. 34, n. 2 [Accessed 24 June 2021] , pp. 221-229. https://doi.org/10.1590/fst.2014.0050.

160. ung, S. M., Haddad, E. H., Kaur, A., Sirirat, R., Kim, A. Y., Oda, K., Rajaram, S., & Sabaté, J. (2021). A Non-Probiotic Fermented Soy Product Reduces Total and LDL Cholesterol: A Randomized Controlled Crossover Trial. Nutrients, 13(2), 535. https://doi.org/10.3390/nu13020535

161. Yamamoto, S., Sobue, T., Kobayashi, M., Sasaki, S., Tsugane, S., & Japan Public Health Center-Based Prospective Study on Cancer Cardiovascular Diseases Group (2003). Soy, isoflavones, and breast cancer risk in Japan. Journal of the National Cancer Institute, 95(12), 906–913. https://doi.org/10.1093/jnci/95.12.906

162. Fujita, Y., Iki, M., Tamaki, J., Kouda, K., Yura, A., Kadowaki, E., Sato, Y., Moon, J. S., Tomioka, K., Okamoto, N., & Kurumatani, N. (2012). Association between vitamin K intake from fermented soybeans, natto, and bone mineral density in elderly Japanese men: the Fujiwara-kyo Osteoporosis Risk in Men (FORMEN) study. Osteoporosis international : a journal established as result of cooperation between the European Foundation for Osteoporosis and the National Osteoporosis Foundation of the USA, 23(2), 705–714. https://doi.org/10.1007/s00198-011-1594-1

163. Katsuyama, H., Ideguchi, S., Fukunaga, M., Saijoh, K., & Sunami, S. (2002). Usual dietary intake of fermented soybeans (Natto) is associated with bone mineral density in premenopausal women. Journal of nutritional science and vitaminology, 48(3), 207–215. https://doi.org/10.3177/jnsv.48.207

164. Ikeda, Y., Iki, M., Morita, A., Kajita, E., Kagamimori, S., Kagawa, Y., & Yoneshima, H. (2006). Intake of fermented soybeans, natto, is associated with reduced bone loss in postmenopausal women: Japanese Population-Based Osteoporosis (JPOS) Study. The Journal of nutrition, 136(5), 1323–1328. https://doi.org/10.1093/jn/136.5.1323

165. Yan, F. F., Wang, W. C., & Cheng, H. W. (2020). Bacillus subtilis-based probiotic promotes bone growth by inhibition of inflammation in broilers subjected to cyclic heating episodes. Poultry science, 99(11), 5252–5260. https://doi.org/10.1016/j.psj.2020.08.051

166. Raak, C., Ostermann, T., Boehm, K., & Molsberger, F. (2014). Regular consumption of sauerkraut and its effect on human health: a bibliometric analysis. Global advances in health and medicine, 3(6), 12–18. https://doi.org/10.7453/gahmj.2014.038

167. Swain, M. R., Anandharaj, M., Ray, R. C., & Parveen Rani, R. (2014). Fermented fruits and vegetables of Asia: a potential source of probiotics. Biotechnology research international, 2014, 250424. https://doi.org/10.1155/2014/250424

168. Sharp, M. D., McMahon, D. J., & Broadbent, J. R. (2008). Comparative evaluation of yogurt and low-fat cheddar cheese as delivery media for probiotic Lactobacillus casei. Journal of food science, 73(7), M375–M377. https://doi.org/10.1111/j.1750-3841.2008.00882.x

169. Phillips, M., Kailasapathy, K., & Tran, L. (2006). Viability of commercial probiotic cultures (L. acidophilus, Bifidobacterium sp., L. casei, L. paracasei and L. rhamnosus) in cheddar cheese. International journal of food microbiology, 108(2), 276–280. https://doi.org/10.1016/j.ijfoodmicro.2005.12.009

170. Choi, J., Lee, S. I., Rackerby, B., Goddik, L., Frojen, R., Ha, S. D., Kim, J. H., & Park, S. H. (2020). Microbial communities of a variety of cheeses and comparison between core and rind region of cheeses. Journal of dairy science, 103(5), 4026–4042. https://doi.org/10.3168/jds.2019-17455

171. Jeon, E. B., Son, S. H., Jeewanthi, R., Lee, N. K., & Paik, H. D. (2016). Characterization of Lactobacillus plantarum Lb41, an isolate from kimchi and its application as a probiotic in cottage cheese. Food science and biotechnology, 25(4), 1129–1133. https://doi.org/10.1007/s10068-016-0181-9

172. Heller K. J. (2001). Probiotic bacteria in fermented foods: product characteristics and starter organisms. The American journal of clinical nutrition, 73(2 Suppl), 374S–379S. https://doi.org/10.1093/ajcn/73.2.374s

173. Ganesan, B., Weimer, B. C., Pinzon, J., Dao Kong, N., Rompato, G., Brothersen, C., & McMahon, D. J. (2014). Probiotic bacteria survive in Cheddar cheese and modify populations of other lactic acid bacteria. Journal of applied microbiology, 116(6), 1642–1656. https://doi.org/10.1111/jam.12482

174. Li, J., Zheng, Y., Xu, H., Xi, X., Hou, Q., Feng, S., Wuri, L., Bian, Y., Yu, Z., Kwok, L. Y., Sun, Z., & Sun, T. (2017). Bacterial microbiota of Kazakhstan cheese revealed by single molecule real time (SMRT) sequencing and its comparison with Belgian, Kalmykian and Italian artisanal cheeses. BMC microbiology, 17(1), 13. https://doi.org/10.1186/s12866-016-0911-4

175. Ortakci, F., Broadbent, J. R., McManus, W. R., & McMahon, D. J. (2012). Survival of microencapsulated probiotic Lactobacillus paracasei LBC-1e during manufacture of Mozzarella cheese and simulated gastric digestion. Journal of dairy science, 95(11), 6274–6281. https://doi.org/10.3168/jds.2012-5476

176. Summer, A., Formaggioni, P., Franceschi, P., Di Frangia, F., Righi, F., & Malacarne, M. (2017). Cheese as Functional Food: The Example of Parmigiano Reggiano and Grana Padano. Food technology and biotechnology, 55(3), 277–289. https://doi.org/10.17113/ftb.55.03.17.5233

177. Succi, M., Tremonte, P., Reale, A., Sorrentino, E., Grazia, L., Pacifico, S., & Coppola, R. (2005). Bile salt and acid tolerance of Lactobacillus rhamnosus strains isolated from Parmigiano Reggiano cheese. FEMS microbiology letters, 244(1), 129–137. https://doi.org/10.1016/j.femsle.2005.01.037

178. Moser, A., Schafroth, K., Meile, L., Egger, L., Badertscher, R., & Irmler, S. (2018). Population Dynamics of Lactobacillus helveticus in Swiss Gruyère-Type Cheese Manufactured with Natural Whey Cultures. Frontiers in microbiology, 9, 637. https://doi.org/10.3389/fmicb.2018.00637

179. Bottari, B., Quartieri, A., Prandi, B., Raimondi, S., Leonardi, A., Rossi, M., Ulrici, A., Gatti, M., Sforza, S., Nocetti, M., & Amaretti, A. (2017). Characterization of the peptide fraction from digested Parmigiano Reggiano cheese and its effect on growth of lactobacilli and bifidobacteria. International journal of food microbiology, 255, 32–41. http://doi.org/10.1016/j.ijfoodmicro.2017.05.015

180. Saksena, R., Deepak, D., Khare, A., Sahai, R., Tripathi, L. M., & Srivastava, V. M. (1999). A novel pentasaccharide from the immunostimulant oligosaccharide fraction of buffalo milk. Biochimica et biophysica acta, 1428(2-3), 433–445. https://doi.org/10.1016/s0304-4165(99)00089-6

181. Annamaria Ricciardi, Giuseppe Blaiotta, Alessandro Di Cerbo, Mariantonietta Succi, Maria Aponte,

182. Choi, J., Lee, S. I., Rackerby, B., Goddik, L., Frojen, R., Ha, S. D., Kim, J. H., & Park, S. H. (2020). Microbial communities of a variety of cheeses and comparison between core and rind region of cheeses. Journal of dairy science, 103(5), 4026–4042. https://doi.org/10.3168/jds.2019-17455

183. Moser, A., Schafroth, K., Meile, L., Egger, L., Badertscher, R., & Irmler, S. (2018). Population Dynamics of Lactobacillus helveticus in Swiss Gruyère-Type Cheese Manufactured with Natural Whey Cultures. Frontiers in microbiology, 9, 637. https://doi.org/10.3389/fmicb.2018.00637

184. Denter, J., & Bisping, B. (1994). Formation of B-vitamins by bacteria during the soaking process of soybeans for tempe fermentation. International journal of food microbiology, 22(1), 23–31. https://doi.org/10.1016/0168-1605(94)90004-3

185. Huang, Y.-C., Wu, B.-H., Chu, Y.-L., Chang, W.-C., & Wu, M.-C. (2018). Effects of Tempeh Fermentation with Lactobacillus plantarum and Rhizopus oligosporus on Streptozotocin-Induced Type II Diabetes Mellitus in Rats. Nutrients, 10(9), 1143. doi:10.3390/nu10091143

186. Kumar, R. A. V. I. N. D. E. R., Kaur, M. A. N. P. R. E. E. T., Garsa, A. K., Shrivastava, B. H. U. V. N. E. S. H., Reddy, V. P., & Tyagi, A. (2015). Natural and cultured buttermilk. Fermented milk and dairy products, 203-225. https://www.researchgate.net/profile/Ravinder-Kumar-39/publication/280136366_Natural_and_Cultured_Buttermilk/links/55f696a508ae1d98039770ed/Natural-and-Cultured-Buttermilk.pdf

187. MilkFacts. (n.d.). Yogurt production. Milk facts. http://www.milkfacts.info/Milk%20Processing/Yogurt%20Production.htm#:-:text=The%20main%20(starter)%20cultures%20in,that%20is%20characteristic%20of%20yogurt

188. Aziz Homayouni, Aslan Azizi, Mina Javadi, Solmaz Mahdipour and Hanie Ejtahed, 2012. Factors Influencing Probiotic Survival in Ice Cream: A Review. International Journal of Dairy Science, 7: 1-10, DOI: 10.3923/ijds.2012.1.10

189. Engen, P. A., Green, S. J., Voigt, R. M., Forsyth, C. B., & Keshavarzian, A. (2015). The Gastrointestinal Microbiome: Alcohol Effects on the Composition of Intestinal Microbiota. Alcohol research : current reviews, 37(2), 223–236.

190. Osna, N. A., Donohue, T. M., Jr, & Kharbanda, K. K. (2017). Alcoholic Liver Disease: Pathogenesis and Current Management. Alcohol research : current reviews, 38(2), 147–161.

191. World Health Organization. (2018). Global status report on alcohol and health 2018. World Health Organization. https://www.who.int/publications/i/item/9789241565639

192. Engen, P. A., Green, S. J., Voigt, R. M., Forsyth, C. B., & Keshavarzian, A. (2015). The Gastrointestinal Microbiome: Alcohol Effects on the Composition of Intestinal Microbiota. Alcohol research : current reviews, 37(2), 223–236.

193. Queipo-Ortuño, M. I., Boto-Ordóñez, M., Murri, M., Gomez-Zumaquero, J. M., Clemente-Postigo, M., Estruch, R., Cardona Diaz, F., Andrés-Lacueva, C., & Tinahones, F. J. (2012). Influence of red wine polyphenols and ethanol on the gut microbiota ecology and biochemical biomarkers. The American journal of clinical nutrition, 95(6), 1323–1334. https://doi.org/10.3945/ajcn.111.027847

194. Stivala, L. A., Savio, M., Carafoli, F., Perucca, P., Bianchi, L., Maga, G., Forti, L., Pagnoni, U. M., Albini, A., Prosperi, E., & Vannini, V. (2001). Specific structural determinants are responsible for the antioxidant activity and the cell cycle effects of resveratrol. The Journal of biological chemistry, 276(25), 22586–22594. https://doi.org/10.1074/jbc.M101846200

195. Tzounis, X., Rodriguez-Mateos, A., Vulevic, J., Gibson, G. R., Kwik-Uribe, C., & Spencer, J. P. (2011). Prebiotic evaluation of cocoa-derived flavanols in healthy humans by using a randomized, controlled, double-blind, crossover intervention study. The American journal of clinical nutrition, 93(1), 62–72. https://doi.org/10.3945/ajcn.110.000075

196. Moreno-Arribas, M. V., Bartolomé, B., Peñalvo, J. L., Pérez-Matute, P., & Motilva, M. J. (2020). Relationship between Wine Consumption, Diet and Microbiome Modulation in Alzheimer's Disease. Nutrients, 12(10), 3082. https://doi.org/10.3390/nu12103082

197. Mutlu, E. A., Gillevet, P. M., Rangwala, H., Sikaroodi, M., Naqvi, A., Engen, P. A., Kwasny, M., Lau, C. K., & Keshavarzian, A. (2012). Colonic microbiome is altered in alcoholism. American journal of physiology. Gastrointestinal and liver physiology, 302(9), G966–G978. https://doi.org/10.1152/ajpgi.00380.2011

198. Phillips M. L. (2009). Gut reaction: environmental effects on the human microbiota. Environmental health perspectives, 117(5), A198–A205. https://doi.org/10.1289/ehp.117-a198

199. Langdon, A., Crook, N., & Dantas, G. (2016). The effects of antibiotics on the microbiome throughout development and alternative approaches for therapeutic modulation. Genome medicine, 8(1), 39. https://doi.org/10.1186/s13073-016-0294-z

200. CDC. (2021, March 2). Biggest Threats and Data. Antibiotic / Antimicrobial Resistance (AR / AMR). https://www.cdc.gov/drugresistance/biggest-threats.html

201. World Health Organization. (2020, October 13). Antimicrobial resistance. Antimicrobial resistance. https://www.who.int/news-room/fact-sheets/detail/antimicrobial-resistance

202. de Kraker MEA, Stewardson AJ, Harbarth S (2016) Will 10 Million People Die a Year due to Antimicrobial Resistance by 2050? PLoS Med 13(11): e1002184. https://doi.org/10.1371/journal.pmed.1002184

203. Martin, M. J., Thottathil, S. E., & Newman, T. B. (2015). Antibiotics Overuse in Animal Agriculture: A Call to Action for Health Care Providers. American journal of public health, 105(12), 2409–2410. https://doi.org/10.2105/AJPH.2015.302870

204. Van Boeckel, T. P., Brower, C., Gilbert, M., Grenfell, B. T., Levin, S. A., Robinson, T. P., Teillant, A., & Laxminarayan, R. (2015). Global trends in antimicrobial use in food animals. Proceedings of the National Academy of Sciences of the United States of America, 112(18), 5649–5654. https://doi.org/10.1073/pnas.1503141112

205. Tyrrell, C., Burgess, C. M., Brennan, F. P., & Walsh, F. (2019). Antibiotic resistance in grass and soil. Biochemical Society transactions, 47(1), 477–486. https://doi.org/10.1042/BST20180552

206. Treiber, F. M., & Beranek-Knauer, H. (2021). Antimicrobial Residues in Food from Animal Origin-A Review of the Literature Focusing on Products Collected in Stores and Markets Worldwide. Antibiotics (Basel, Switzerland), 10(5), 534. https://doi.org/10.3390/antibiotics10050534

207. Branch, J. (2019, September 12). What Do You Really Get When You Buy Organic? Health. https://www.consumerreports.org/organic-foods/what-do-you-really-get-when-you-buy-organic/

208. Nhung, N. T., Van, N., Cuong, N. V., Duong, T., Nhat, T. T., Hang, T., Nhi, N., Kiet, B. T., Hien, V. B., Ngoc, P. T., Campbell, J., Thwaites, G., & Carrique-Mas, J. (2018). Antimicrobial residues and resistance against critically important antimicrobials in non-typhoidal Salmonella from meat sold at wet markets and supermarkets in Vietnam. International journal of food microbiology, 266, 301–309. https://doi.org/10.1016/j.ijfoodmicro.2017.12.015

209. Jansomboon, W., Boontanon, S. K., Boontanon, N., Polprasert, C., & Thi Da, C. (2016). Monitoring and determination of sulfonamide antibiotics (sulfamethoxydiazine, sulfamethazine, sulfamethoxazole and sulfadiazine) in imported Pangasius catfish products in Thailand using liquid chromatography coupled with tandem mass spectrometry. Food chemistry, 212, 635–640. https://doi.org/10.1016/j.foodchem.2016.06.026

210. Palaniyappan, V., Nagalingam, A. K., Ranganathan, H. P., Kandhikuppam, K. B., Kothandam, H. P., & Vasu, S. (2013). Antibiotics in South Indian coastal sea and farmed prawns (Penaeus monodon). Food additives & contaminants. Part B, Surveillance, 6(3), 196–199. https://doi.org/10.1080/19393210.2013.787555

211. Liu, X., Steele, J. C., & Meng, X. Z. (2017). Usage, residue, and human health risk of antibiotics in Chinese aquaculture: A review. Environmental pollution (Barking, Essex : 1987), 223, 161–169. https://doi.org/10.1016/j.envpol.2017.01.003

212. Zhang, R., Pei, J., Zhang, R., Wang, S., Zeng, W., Huang, D., Wang, Y., Zhang, Y., Wang, Y., & Yu, K. (2018). Occurrence and distribution of antibiotics in mariculture farms, estuaries and the coast of the Beibu Gulf, China: Bioconcentration and diet safety of seafood. Ecotoxicology and environmental safety, 154, 27–35. https://doi.org/10.1016/j.ecoenv.2018.02.006

213. Calvo, T., & Melzer-Warren, R. (2020, September 10). What 'No Antibiotics' Claims Really Mean. Overuse of Antibiotics. https://www.consumerreports.org/overuse-of-antibiotics/what-no-antibiotic-claims-really-mean/

214. World health organization. (2020, July 31). Antibiotic resistance. Antibiotic resistance. https://www.who.int/news-room/fact-sheets/detail/antibiotic-resistance

215. Ruiz-Ojeda, F. J., Plaza-Díaz, J., Sáez-Lara, M. J., & Gil, A. (2019). Effects of Sweeteners on the Gut Microbiota: A Review of Experimental Studies and Clinical Trials. Advances in nutrition (Bethesda, Md.), 10(suppl_1), S31–S48. https://doi.org/10.1093/advances/nmy037

216. Bian, X., Chi, L., Gao, B., Tu, P., Ru, H., & Lu, K. (2017). The artificial sweetener acesulfame potassium affects the gut microbiome and body weight gain in CD-1 mice. PloS one, 12(6), e0178426. https://doi.org/10.1371/journal.pone.0178426

217. Ahmad, S. Y., Friel, J., & Mackay, D. (2020). The Effects of Non-Nutritive Artificial Sweeteners, Aspartame and Sucralose, on the Gut Microbiome in Healthy Adults: Secondary Outcomes of a Randomized Double-Blinded Crossover Clinical Trial. Nutrients, 12(11), 3408. https://doi.org/10.3390/nu12113408

218. Pepino, M. Y., & Bourne, C. (2011). Non-nutritive sweeteners, energy balance, and glucose homeostasis. Current opinion in clinical nutrition and metabolic care, 14(4), 391–395. https://doi.org/10.1097/MCO.0b013e3283468e7e

219. Choudhary, A. K., & Pretorius, E. (2017). Revisiting the safety of aspartame. Nutrition reviews, 75(9), 718–730. https://doi.org/10.1093/nutrit/nux035

220. Amin, K. A., Al-muzafar, H. M., & Abd Elsttar, A. H. (2016). Effect of sweetener and flavoring agent on oxidative indices, liver and kidney function levels in rats. Indian journal of experimental biology, 54(1), 56–63.

221. Azeez, O. H., Alkass, S. Y., & Persike, D. S. (2019). Long-Term Saccharin Consumption and Increased Risk of Obesity, Diabetes, Hepatic Dysfunction, and Renal Impairment in Rats. Medicina (Kaunas, Lithuania), 55(10), 681. https://doi.org/10.3390/medicina55100681

222. Pepino, M. Y., Tiemann, C. D., Patterson, B. W., Wice, B. M., & Klein, S. (2013). Sucralose affects glycemic and hormonal responses to an oral glucose load. Diabetes care, 36(9), 2530–2535. https://doi.org/10.2337/dc12-2221

223. Romo-Romo, A., Aguilar-Salinas, C. A., Brito-Córdova, G. X., Gómez-Díaz, R. A., & Almeda-Valdes, P. (2018). Sucralose decreases insulin sensitivity in healthy subjects: a randomized controlled trial. The American journal of clinical nutrition, 108(3), 485–491. https://doi.org/10.1093/ajcn/nqy152

224. Lertrit, A., Srimachai, S., Saetung, S., Chanprasertyothin, S., Chailurkit, L. O., Areevut, C., Katekao, P., Ongphiphadhanakul, B., & Sriphrapradang, C. (2018). Effects of sucralose on insulin and glucagon-like peptide-1 secretion in healthy subjects: a randomized, double-blind, placebo-controlled trial. Nutrition (Burbank, Los Angeles County, Calif.), 55-56, 125–130. https://doi.org/10.1016/j.nut.2018.04.001

225. Young, D. A., & Bowen, W. H. (1990). The influence of sucralose on bacterial metabolism. Journal of dental research, 69(8), 1480–1484. https://doi.org/10.1177/00220345900690080601

226. Omran, A., Ahearn, G., Bowers, D., Swenson, J., & Coughlin, C. (2013). Metabolic effects of sucralose on environmental bacteria. Journal of toxicology, 2013, 372986. https://doi.org/10.1155/2013/372986

227. Abou-Donia, M. B., El-Masry, E. M., Abdel-Rahman, A. A., McLendon, R. E., & Schiffman, S. S. (2008). Splenda alters gut microflora and increases intestinal p-glycoprotein and cytochrome p-450 in male rats. Journal of toxicology and environmental health. Part A, 71(21), 1415–1429. https://doi.org/10.1080/15287390802328630

228. Samuel, P., Ayoob, K. T., Magnuson, B. A., Wölwer-Rieck, U., Jeppesen, P. B., Rogers, P. J., Rowland, I., & Mathews, R. (2018). Stevia Leaf to Stevia Sweetener: Exploring Its Science, Benefits, and Future Potential. The Journal of nutrition, 148(7), 1186S–1205S. https://doi.org/10.1093/jn/nxy102

229. Sanches Lopes, S. M., Francisco, M. G., Higashi, B., de Almeida, R., Krausová, G., Pilau, E. J., Gonçalves, J. E., Gonçalves, R., & Oliveira, A. (2016). Chemical characterization and prebiotic activity of fructo-oligosaccharides from Stevia rebaudiana (Bertoni) roots and in vitro adventitious root cultures. Carbohydrate polymers, 152, 718–725. https://doi.org/10.1016/j.carbpol.2016.07.043

230. Ruiz-Ojeda, F. J., Plaza-Díaz, J., Sáez-Lara, M. J., & Gil, A. (2019). Effects of Sweeteners on the Gut Microbiota: A Review of Experimental Studies and Clinical Trials. Advances in nutrition (Bethesda, Md.), 10(suppl_1), S31–S48. https://doi.org/10.1093/advances/nmy037

231. Melis, M. S., Rocha, S. T., & Augusto, A. (2009). Steviol effect, a glycoside of Stevia rebaudiana, on glucose clearances in rats. Brazilian journal of biology = Revista brasileira de biologia, 69(2), 371–374. https://doi.org/10.1590/s1519-69842009000200019

232. Yan, T., Wang, H., Cao, L., Wang, Q., Takahashi, S., Yagai, T., Li, G., Krausz, K. W., Wang, G., Gonzalez, F. J., & Hao, H. (2018). Glycyrrhizin Alleviates Nonalcoholic Steatohepatitis via Modulating Bile Acids and Meta-Inflammation. Drug metabolism and disposition: the biological fate of chemicals, 46(9), 1310–1319. https://doi.org/10.1124/dmd.118.082008

233. Roohbakhsh, A., Iranshahy, M., & Iranshahi, M. (2016). Glycyrrhetinic Acid and Its Derivatives: Anti-Cancer and Cancer Chemopreventive Properties, Mechanisms of Action and Structure- Cytotoxic Activity Relationship. Current medicinal chemistry, 23(5), 498–517. https://doi.org/10.2174/0929867323666160112122256

234. Cinatl, J., Morgenstern, B., Bauer, G., Chandra, P., Rabenau, H., & Doerr, H. W. (2003). Glycyrrhizin, an active component of liquorice roots, and replication of SARS-associated coronavirus. Lancet (London, England), 361(9374), 2045–2046. https://doi.org/10.1016/s0140-6736(03)13615-x

235. Bailly, C., & Vergoten, G. (2020). Glycyrrhizin: An alternative drug for the treatment of COVID-19 infection and the associated respiratory syndrome?. Pharmacology & therapeutics, 214, 107618. https://doi.org/10.1016/j.pharmthera.2020.107618

236. Chrzanowski, J., Chrzanowska, A., & Graboń, W. (2021). Glycyrrhizin: An old weapon against a novel coronavirus. Phytotherapy research : PTR, 35(2), 629–636. https://doi.org/10.1002/ptr.6852

237. Ruiz-Ojeda, F. J., Plaza-Díaz, J., Sáez-Lara, M. J., & Gil, A. (2019). Effects of Sweeteners on the Gut Microbiota: A Review of Experimental Studies and Clinical Trials. Advances in nutrition (Bethesda, Md.), 10(suppl_1), S31–S48. https://doi.org/10.1093/advances/nmy037

238. Zhou, G., Zhang, Y., Li, Y., Wang, M., & Li, X. (2018). The metabolism of a natural product mogroside V, in healthy and type 2 diabetic rats. Journal of chromatography. B, Analytical technologies in the biomedical and life sciences, 1079, 25–33. https://doi.org/10.1016/j.jchromb.2018.02.002

239. Xu, F., Li, D. P., Huang, Z. C., Lu, F. L., Wang, L., Huang, Y. L., Wang, R. F., Liu, G. X., Shang, M. Y., & Cai, S. Q. (2015). Exploring in vitro, in vivo metabolism of mogroside V and distribution of its metabolites in rats by HPLC-ESI-IT-TOF-MS(n). Journal of pharmaceutical and biomedical analysis, 115, 418–430. https://doi.org/10.1016/j.jpba.2015.07.024

240. Murata, Y., Ogawa, T., Suzuki, Y. A., Yoshikawa, S., Inui, H., Sugiura, M., & Nakano, Y. (2010). Digestion and absorption of Siraitia grosvenori triterpenoids in the rat. Bioscience, biotechnology, and biochemistry, 74(3), 673–676. https://doi.org/10.1271/bbb.90832

241. Zhang, Y., Zhou, G., Peng, Y., Wang, M., & Li, X. (2020). Anti-hyperglycemic and anti-hyperlipidemic effects of a special fraction of Luohanguo extract on obese T2DM rats. Journal of ethnopharmacology, 247, 112273. https://doi.org/10.1016/j.jep.2019.112273

242. Sung, Y. Y., Yuk, H. J., Yang, W. K., Kim, S. H., & Kim, D. S. (2020). Siraitia grosvenorii Residual Extract Attenuates Atopic Dermatitis by Regulating Immune Dysfunction and Skin Barrier Abnormality. Nutrients, 12(12), 3638. https://doi.org/10.3390/nu12123638

243. Gong, X., Chen, N., Ren, K., Jia, J., Wei, K., Zhang, L., Lv, Y., Wang, J., & Li, M. (2019). The Fruits of Siraitia grosvenorii: A Review of a Chinese Food-Medicine. Frontiers in pharmacology, 10, 1400. https://doi.org/10.3389/fphar.2019.01400

244. Li, C., Lin, L. M., Sui, F., Wang, Z. M., Huo, H. R., Dai, L., & Jiang, T. L. (2014). Chemistry and pharmacology of Siraitia grosvenorii: a review. Chinese journal of natural medicines, 12(2), 89–102. https://doi.org/10.1016/S1875-5364(14)60015-7

245. Grembecka M. (2015). Natural sweeteners in a human diet. Roczniki Panstwowego Zakladu Higieny, 66(3), 195–202.

246. Ruiz-Ojeda, F. J., Plaza-Díaz, J., Sáez-Lara, M. J., & Gil, A. (2019). Effects of Sweeteners on the Gut Microbiota: A Review of Experimental Studies and Clinical Trials. Advances in nutrition (Bethesda, Md.), 10(suppl_1), S31–S48. https://doi.org/10.1093/advances/nmy037

247. Gostner, A., Blaut, M., Schäffer, V., Kozianowski, G., Theis, S., Klingeberg, M., Dombrowski, Y., Martin, D., Ehrhardt, S., Taras, D., Schwiertz, A., Kleessen, B., Lührs, H., Schauber, J., Dorbath, D., Menzel, T., & Scheppach, W. (2006). Effect of isomalt consumption on faecal microflora and colonic metabolism in healthy volunteers. The British journal of nutrition, 95(1), 40–50. https://doi.org/10.1079/bjn20051589

248. Małgorzata Grembecka,Sugar Alcohols,Editor(s): Laurence Melton, Fereidoon Shahidi, Peter Varelis,

249. Beards, E., Tuohy, K., & Gibson, G. (2010). A human volunteer study to assess the impact of confectionery sweeteners on the gut microbiota composition. The British journal of nutrition, 104(5), 701–708. https://doi.org/10.1017/S0007114510001078

250. Chen, M., Zhang, W., Wu, H., Guang, C., & Mu, W. (2020). Mannitol: physiological functionalities, determination methods, biotechnological production, and applications. Applied microbiology and biotechnology, 104(16), 6941–6951. https://doi.org/10.1007/s00253-020-10757-y

251. Salminen, S., Salminen, E., Koivistoinen, P., Bridges, J., & Marks, V. (1985). Gut microflora interactions with xylitol in the mouse, rat and man. Food and chemical toxicology : an international journal published for the British Industrial Biological Research Association, 23(11), 985–990. https://doi.org/10.1016/0278-6915(85)90248-0

252. Naaber, P., Mikelsaar, R. H., Salminen, S., & Mikelsaar, M. (1998). Bacterial translocation, intestinal microflora and morphological changes of intestinal mucosa in experimental models of Clostridium difficile infection. Journal of medical microbiology, 47(7), 591–598. https://doi.org/10.1099/00222615-47-7-591

253. Do, M. H., Lee, E., Oh, M. J., Kim, Y., & Park, H. Y. (2018). High-Glucose or -Fructose Diet Cause Changes of the Gut Microbiota and Metabolic Disorders in Mice without Body Weight Change. Nutrients, 10(6), 761. https://doi.org/10.3390/nu10060761

254. Lana P. Franco, Carla C. Morais, Cristiane Cominetti, Normal-weight obesity syndrome: diagnosis, prevalence, and clinical implications, Nutrition Reviews, Volume 74, Issue 9, September 2016, Pages 558–570, https://doi.org/10.1093/nutrit/nuw019

255. Satokari R. (2020). High Intake of Sugar and the Balance between Pro- and Anti-Inflammatory Gut Bacteria. Nutrients, 12(5), 1348. https://doi.org/10.3390/nu12051348

256. Zhang, M., & Yang, X. J. (2016). Effects of a high fat diet on intestinal microbiota and gastrointestinal diseases. World journal of gastroenterology, 22(40), 8905–8909. https://doi.org/10.3748/wjg.v22.i40.8905

257. Hua, Y., Fan, R., Zhao, L., Tong, C., Qian, X., Zhang, M., Xiao, R., & Ma, W. (2020). Trans-fatty acids alter the gut microbiota in high-fat-diet-induced obese rats. The British journal of nutrition, 124(12), 1251–1263. https://doi.org/10.1017/S0007114520001841

258. Muniz, L. B., Alves-Santos, A. M., Camargo, F., Martins, D. B., Celes, M., & Naves, M. (2019). High-Lard and High-Cholesterol Diet, but not High-Lard Diet, Leads to Metabolic Disorders in a Modified Dyslipidemia Model. Arquivos brasileiros de cardiologia, 113(5), 896–902. https://doi.org/10.5935/abc.20190149

259. Shao, S. S., Zhao, Y. F., Song, Y. F., Xu, C., Yang, J. M., Xuan, S. M., Yan, H. L., Yu, C. X., Zhao, M., Xu, J., & Zhao, J. J. (2014). Dietary high-fat lard intake induces thyroid dysfunction and abnormal morphology in rats. Acta pharmacologica Sinica, 35(11), 1411–1420. https://doi.org/10.1038/aps.2014.82

260. Just, S., Mondot, S., Ecker, J., Wegner, K., Rath, E., Gau, L., Streidl, T., Hery-Arnaud, G., Schmidt, S., Lesker, T. R., Bieth, V., Dunkel, A., Strowig, T., Hofmann, T., Haller, D., Liebisch, G., Gérard, P., Rohn, S., Lepage, P., & Clavel, T. (2018). The gut

microbiota drives the impact of bile acids and fat source in diet on mouse metabolism. Microbiome, 6(1), 134. https://doi.org/10.1186/s40168-018-0510-8

261. Yan, S., Zhou, H., Liu, S., Wang, J., Zeng, Y., Matias, F. B., & Wen, L. (2020). Differential effects of Chinese high-fat dietary habits on lipid metabolism: mechanisms and health implications. Lipids in health and disease, 19(1), 30. https://doi.org/10.1186/s12944-020-01212-y

262. Muniz, L. B., Alves-Santos, A. M., Camargo, F., Martins, D. B., Celes, M., & Naves, M. (2019). High-Lard and High-Cholesterol Diet, but not High-Lard Diet, Leads to Metabolic Disorders in a Modified Dyslipidemia Model. Arquivos brasileiros de cardiologia, 113(5), 896–902. https://doi.org/10.5935/abc.20190149

263. Wang, J., Wang, X., Li, J., Chen, Y., Yang, W., & Zhang, L. (2015). Effects of Dietary Coconut Oil as a Medium-chain Fatty Acid Source on Performance, Carcass Composition and Serum Lipids in Male Broilers. Asian-Australasian journal of animal sciences, 28(2), 223–230. https://doi.org/10.5713/ajas.14.0328

264. Rial, S. A., Karelis, A. D., Bergeron, K. F., & Mounier, C. (2016). Gut Microbiota and Metabolic Health: The Potential Beneficial Effects of a Medium Chain Triglyceride Diet in Obese Individuals. Nutrients, 8(5), 281. https://doi.org/10.3390/nu8050281

265. Dayrit, F. M. (2014). Lauric acid is a medium-chain fatty acid, coconut oil is a medium-chain triglyceride. Philippine Journal of Science, 143(2), 157-166.

266. Oteng, A. B., & Kersten, S. (2020). Mechanisms of Action of trans Fatty Acids. Advances in nutrition (Bethesda, Md.), 11(3), 697–708. https://doi.org/10.1093/advances/nmz125

267. Guillaume C., et al. "Evaluation of Chemical and Physical Changes in Different Commercial Oils during Heating". Acta Scientific Nutritional Health

268. Gorzynik-Debicka, M., Przychodzen, P., Cappello, F., Kuban-Jankowska, A., Marino Gammazza, A., Knap, N., Wozniak, M., & Gorska-Ponikowska, M. (2018). Potential Health Benefits of Olive Oil and Plant Polyphenols. International journal of molecular sciences, 19(3), 686. https://doi.org/10.3390/ijms19030686

269. Unhapipatpong, C., Shantavasinkul, P. C., Kasemsup, V., Siriyotha, S., Warodomwichit, D., Maneesuwannarat, S., Vathesatogkit, P., Sritara, P., & Thakkinstian, A. (2021). Tropical Oil Consumption and Cardiovascular Disease: An Umbrella Review of Systematic Reviews and Meta Analyses. Nutrients, 13(5), 1549. https://doi.org/10.3390/nu13051549

270. Tong, Y., Gao, H., Qi, Q., Liu, X., Li, J., Gao, J., Li, P., Wang, Y., Du, L., & Wang, C. (2021). High fat diet, gut microbiome and gastrointestinal cancer. Theranostics, 11(12), 5889–5910. https://doi.org/10.7150/thno.56157

271. Ibiebele, T. I., Hughes, M. C., Whiteman, D. C., Webb, P. M., & Australian Cancer Study (2012). Dietary patterns and risk of esophageal cancers: a population-based case-control study. The British journal of nutrition, 107(8), 1207–1216. https://doi.org/10.1017/S0007114511004247

272. Ang, Q. Y., Alexander, M., Newman, J. C., Tian, Y., Cai, J., Upadhyay, V., Turnbaugh, J. A., Verdin, E., Hall, K. D., Leibel, R. L., Ravussin, E., Rosenbaum, M., Patterson, A. D., & Turnbaugh, P. J. (2020). Ketogenic Diets Alter the Gut Microbiome, Resulting in Decreased Intestinal Th17 Cells. Cell, 181(6), 1263–1275.e16. https://doi.org/10.1016/j.cell.2020.04.027

273. Grandl, G., Straub, L., Rudigier, C., Arnold, M., Wueest, S., Konrad, D., & Wolfrum, C. (2018). Short-term feeding of a ketogenic diet induces more severe hepatic insulin resistance than an obesogenic high-fat diet. The Journal of physiology, 596(19), 4597–4609. https://doi.org/10.1113/JP275173

274. Selmin, O. I., Papoutsis, A. J., Hazan, S., Smith, C., Greenfield, N., Donovan, M. G., Wren, S. N., Doetschman, T. C., Snider, J. M., Snider, A. J., Chow, S. H., & Romagnolo, D. F. (2021). n-6 High Fat Diet Induces Gut Microbiome Dysbiosis and Colonic Inflammation. International journal of molecular sciences, 22(13), 6919. https://doi.org/10.3390/ijms22136919

275. Cândido, F. G., Valente, F. X., Grześkowiak, Ł. M., Moreira, A., Rocha, D., & Alfenas, R. (2018). Impact of dietary fat on gut microbiota and low-grade systemic inflammation: mechanisms and clinical implications on obesity. International journal of food sciences and nutrition, 69(2), 125–143. https://doi.org/10.1080/09637486.2017.1343286

276. Jamar, G., Ribeiro, D. A., & Pisani, L. P. (2021). High-fat or high-sugar diets as trigger inflammation in the microbiota-gut-brain axis. Critical reviews in food science and nutrition, 61(5), 836–854. https://doi.org/10.1080/10408398.2020.1747046

277. Costantini, L., Molinari, R., Farinon, B., & Merendino, N. (2017). Impact of Omega-3 Fatty Acids on the Gut Microbiota. International journal of molecular sciences, 18(12), 2645. https://doi.org/10.3390/ijms18122645

278. Fu, Y., Wang, Y., Gao, H., Li, D., Jiang, R., Ge, L., Tong, C., & Xu, K. (2021). Associations among Dietary Omega-3 Polyunsaturated Fatty Acids, the Gut Microbiota, and Intestinal Immunity. Mediators of inflammation, 2021, 8879227. https://doi.org/10.1155/2021/8879227

279. Fu, Y., Wang, Y., Gao, H., Li, D., Jiang, R., Ge, L., Tong, C., & Xu, K. (2021). Associations among Dietary Omega-3 Polyunsaturated Fatty Acids, the Gut Microbiota, and Intestinal Immunity. Mediators of inflammation, 2021, 8879227. https://doi.org/10.1155/2021/8879227

280. Shahidi, F., & Ambigaipalan, P. (2018). Omega-3 Polyunsaturated Fatty Acids and Their Health Benefits. Annual review of food science and technology, 9, 345–381. https://doi.org/10.1146/annurev-food-111317-095850

281. Adarme-Vega, T. C., Lim, D. K., Timmins, M., Vernen, F., Li, Y., & Schenk, P. M. (2012). Microalgal biofactories: a promising approach towards sustainable omega-3 fatty acid production. Microbial cell factories, 11, 96. https://doi.org/10.1186/1475-2859-11-96

282. Fu, Y., Wang, Y., Gao, H., Li, D., Jiang, R., Ge, L., Tong, C., & Xu, K. (2021). Associations among Dietary Omega-3 Polyunsaturated Fatty Acids, the Gut Microbiota, and Intestinal Immunity. Mediators of inflammation, 2021, 8879227. https://doi.org/10.1155/2021/8879227

283. Li, J., Pora, B., Dong, K., & Hasjim, J. (2021). Health benefits of docosahexaenoic acid and its bioavailability: A review. Food science & nutrition, 9(9), 5229–5243. https://doi.org/10.1002/fsn3.2299

284. Kris-Etherton, P. M., Harris, W. S., Appel, L. J., & American Heart Association. Nutrition Committee (2002). Fish consumption, fish oil, omega-3 fatty acids, and cardiovascular disease. Circulation, 106(21), 2747–2757. https://doi.org/10.1161/01.cir.0000038493.65177.94

285. Li, J., Pora, B., Dong, K., & Hasjim, J. (2021). Health benefits of docosahexaenoic acid and its bioavailability: A review. Food science & nutrition, 9(9), 5229–5243. https://doi.org/10.1002/fsn3.2299

286. Shahidi, F., & Ambigaipalan, P. (2018). Omega-3 Polyunsaturated Fatty Acids and Their Health Benefits. Annual review of food science and technology, 9, 345–381. https://doi.org/10.1146/annurev-food-111317-095850

287. Mozaffarian, D., & Wu, J. H. (2012). (n-3) fatty acids and cardiovascular health: are effects of EPA and DHA shared or complementary?. The Journal of nutrition, 142(3), 614S–625S. https://doi.org/10.3945/jn.111.149633

288. Haro, C., García Carpintero, S., Rangel Zúñiga, O. A., Alcalá-Díaz, J. F., Landa, B. B., Clemente, J. C., Pérez-Martinez, P., López-Miranda, J., Pérez-Jiménez, F., & Camargo, A. (2017). Consumption of Two Healthy Dietary Patterns Restored Microbiota Dysbiosis in Obese Patients with Metabolic Dysfunction. Molecular nutrition & food research, 61(12), 10.1002/mnfr.201700300. https://doi.org/10.1002/mnfr.201700300

289. BYJU'S. (n.d.). Pesticides. chemistry. https://byjus.com/chemistry/pesticides/

290. Ruuskanen, S., Rainio, M. J., Gómez-Gallego, C., Selenius, O., Salminen, S., Collado, M. C., Saikkonen, K., Saloniemi, I., & Helander, M. (2020). Glyphosate-based herbicides influence antioxidants, reproductive hormones and gut microbiome but not reproduction: A long-term experiment in an avian model. Environmental pollution (Barking, Essex : 1987), 266(Pt 1), 115108. https://doi.org/10.1016/j.envpol.2020.115108

291. Rueda-Ruzafa, L., Cruz, F., Roman, P., & Cardona, D. (2019). Gut microbiota and neurological effects of glyphosate. Neurotoxicology, 75, 1–8. https://doi.org/10.1016/j.neuro.2019.08.006

292. Mikhail Y. Syromyatnikov & Mariya M. Isuwa & Olga V. Savinkova & Mariya I. Derevshchikova & Vasily N. Popov, 2020. "The Effect of Pesticides on the Microbiome of Animals," Agriculture, MDPI, Open Access Journal, vol. 10(3), pages 1-14, March. https://doi.org/10.3390/agriculture10030079

293. Dill, G. M., Cajacob, C. A., & Padgette, S. R. (2008). Glyphosate-resistant crops: adoption, use and future considerations. Pest management science, 64(4), 326–331. https://doi.org/10.1002/ps.1501

294. IFPS. (n.d.). Price Look Up Codes. PLU CODES. https://www.ifpsglobal.com/PLU-Codes

295. Gallè, F., Valeriani, F., Cattaruzza, M. S., Ubaldi, F., Romano Spica, V., Liguori, G., WDPP, Working Group on Doping Prevention Project, & GSMS-SItI, Working Group on Movement Sciences for Health, Italian Society of Hygiene, Preventive Medicine and Public Health (2019). Exploring the association between physical activity and gut microbiota composition: a review of current evidence. Annali di igiene : medicina preventiva e di comunita, 31(6), 582–589. https://doi.org/10.7416/ai.2019.2318

296. Matenchuk, B. A., Mandhane, P. J., & Kozyrskyj, A. L. (2020). Sleep, circadian rhythm, and gut microbiota. Sleep medicine reviews, 53, 101340. https://doi.org/10.1016/j.smrv.2020.101340

297. Miller W. L. (2018). The Hypothalamic-Pituitary-Adrenal Axis: A Brief History. Hormone research in paediatrics, 89(4), 212–223. https://doi.org/10.1159/000487755

298. Li, Y., Hao, Y., Fan, F., & Zhang, B. (2018). The Role of Microbiome in Insomnia, Circadian Disturbance and Depression. Frontiers in psychiatry, 9, 669. https://doi.org/10.3389/fpsyt.2018.00669

299. Krueger, J. M., & Opp, M. R. (2016). Sleep and Microbes. International review of neurobiology, 131, 207–225. https://doi.org/10.1016/bs.irn.2016.07.003

300. Gui, X., Yang, Z., & Li, M. D. (2021). Effect of Cigarette Smoke on Gut Microbiota: State of Knowledge. Frontiers in physiology, 12, 673341. https://doi.org/10.3389/fphys.2021.673341

301. Galley, J. D., Nelson, M. C., Yu, Z., Dowd, S. E., Walter, J., Kumar, P. S., Lyte, M., & Bailey, M. T. (2014). Exposure to a social stressor disrupts the community structure of the colonic mucosa-associated microbiota. BMC microbiology, 14, 189. https://doi.org/10.1186/1471-2180-14-189

302. Partrick, K. A., Chassaing, B., Beach, L. Q., McCann, K. E., Gewirtz, A. T., & Huhman, K. L. (2018). Acute and repeated exposure to social stress reduces gut microbiota diversity in Syrian hamsters. Behavioural brain research, 345, 39–48. https://doi.org/10.1016/j.bbr.2018.02.005

303. Madison, A., & Kiecolt-Glaser, J. K. (2019). Stress, depression, diet, and the gut microbiota: human-bacteria interactions at the core of psychoneuroimmunology and nutrition. Current opinion in behavioral sciences, 28, 105–110. https://doi.org/10.1016/j.cobeha.2019.01.011

304. Kumar Singh, A., Cabral, C., Kumar, R., Ganguly, R., Kumar Rana, H., Gupta, A., Rosaria Lauro, M., Carbone, C., Reis, F., & Pandey, A. K. (2019). Beneficial Effects of Dietary Polyphenols on Gut Microbiota and Strategies to Improve Delivery Efficiency. Nutrients, 11(9), 2216. https://doi.org/10.3390/nu11092216

305. Kasprzak-Drozd, K., Oniszczuk, T., Stasiak, M., & Oniszczuk, A. (2021). Beneficial Effects of Phenolic Compounds on Gut Microbiota and Metabolic Syndrome. International journal of molecular sciences, 22(7), 3715. https://doi.org/10.3390/ijms22073715

306. Azzini, E., Giacometti, J., & Russo, G. L. (2017). Antiobesity Effects of Anthocyanins in Preclinical and Clinical Studies. Oxidative medicine and cellular longevity, 2017, 2740364. https://doi.org/10.1155/2017/2740364

307. Xiao, J. B., & Högger, P. (2015). Dietary polyphenols and type 2 diabetes: current insights and future perspectives. Current medicinal chemistry, 22(1), 23–38. https://doi.org/10.2174/0929867321666140706130807

308. Khoo, H. E., Azlan, A., Tang, S. T., & Lim, S. M. (2017). Anthocyanidins and anthocyanins: colored pigments as food, pharmaceutical ingredients, and the potential health benefits. Food & nutrition research, 61(1), 1361779. https://doi.org/10.1080/16546628.2017.1361779

309. Hua Zhang, Rong Tsao,Dietary polyphenols, oxidative stress and antioxidant and anti-inflammatory effects,Current Opinion in Food Science,Volume 8,2016,Pages 33-42,

310. Hussain, T., Tan, B., Yin, Y., Blachier, F., Tossou, M. C., & Rahu, N. (2016). Oxidative Stress and Inflammation: What Polyphenols Can Do for Us?. Oxidative medicine and cellular longevity, 2016, 7432797. https://doi.org/10.1155/2016/7432797

311. Afaq, F., & Katiyar, S. K. (2011). Polyphenols: skin photoprotection and inhibition of photocarcinogenesis. Mini reviews in medicinal chemistry, 11(14), 1200–1215. https://doi.org/10.2174/138955711791091200

312. Zhou, Y., Zheng, J., Li, Y., Xu, D. P., Li, S., Chen, Y. M., & Li, H. B. (2016). Natural Polyphenols for Prevention and Treatment of Cancer. Nutrients, 8(8), 515. https://doi.org/10.3390/nu8080515

313. Basu, A., Rhone, M., & Lyons, T. J. (2010). Berries: emerging impact on cardiovascular health. Nutrition reviews, 68(3), 168–177. https://doi.org/10.1111/j.1753-4887.2010.00273.x

314. Catalgol, B., Batirel, S., Taga, Y., & Ozer, N. K. (2012). Resveratrol: French paradox revisited. Frontiers in pharmacology, 3, 141. https://doi.org/10.3389/fphar.2012.00141

315. Laura Marín, Elisa M. Miguélez, Claudio J. Villar, Felipe Lombó, "Bioavailability of Dietary Polyphenols and Gut Microbiota Metabolism: Antimicrobial Properties", BioMed Research International, vol. 2015, Article ID 905215, 18 pages, 2015. https://doi.org/10.1155/2015/905215

316. Dryden, G. W., Song, M., & McClain, C. (2006). Polyphenols and gastrointestinal diseases. Current opinion in gastroenterology, 22(2), 165–170. https://doi.org/10.1097/01.mog.0000208463.69266.8c

317. Field, D. T., Williams, C. M., & Butler, L. T. (2011). Consumption of cocoa flavanols results in an acute improvement in visual and cognitive functions. Physiology & behavior, 103(3-4), 255–260. https://doi.org/10.1016/j.physbeh.2011.02.013

318. Sorond, F. A., Lipsitz, L. A., Hollenberg, N. K., & Fisher, N. D. (2008). Cerebral blood flow response to flavanol-rich cocoa in healthy elderly humans. Neuropsychiatric disease and treatment, 4(2), 433–440.

319. Mehan S, Kaur R, Parveen S, Khanna D, Kalra S. Polyphenol Ellagic Acid-Targeting To Brain: A Hidden Treasure. International Journal of Neurology Research 2015; 1(3): 141-152. http://www.ghrnet.org/index.php/ijnr/article/view/1107

320. Kanti Bhooshan Pandey, Syed Ibrahim Rizvi, "Plant Polyphenols as Dietary Antioxidants in Human Health and Disease", Oxidative Medicine and Cellular Longevity, vol. 2, Article ID 897484, 9 pages, 2009. https://doi.org/10.4161/oxim.2.5.9498

321. Zhou, Y., Zheng, J., Li, Y., Xu, D. P., Li, S., Chen, Y. M., & Li, H. B. (2016). Natural Polyphenols for Prevention and Treatment of Cancer. Nutrients, 8(8), 515. https://doi.org/10.3390/nu8080515

322. Khoo, H. E., Azlan, A., Tang, S. T., & Lim, S. M. (2017). Anthocyanidins and anthocyanins: colored pigments as food, pharmaceutical ingredients, and the potential health benefits. Food & nutrition research, 61(1), 1361779. https://doi.org/10.1080/16546628.2017.1361779

323. Mattioli, R., Francioso, A., Mosca, L., & Silva, P. (2020). Anthocyanins: A Comprehensive Review of Their Chemical Properties and Health Effects on Cardiovascular and Neurodegenerative Diseases. Molecules (Basel, Switzerland), 25(17), 3809. https://doi.org/10.3390/molecules25173809

324. Chen, A. Y., & Chen, Y. C. (2013). A review of the dietary flavonoid, kaempferol on human health and cancer chemoprevention. Food chemistry, 138(4), 2099–2107. https://doi.org/10.1016/j.foodchem.2012.11.139

325. Bender, B. (2018, October 1). 63 Kaempferol Rich Foods (Ranked). https://www.intake.health/post/63-kaempferol-rich-foods-ranked

326. Mughal MH (2019) Turmeric polyphenols: A comprehensive review. Integr Food Nutr Metab 6: DOI: 10.15761/IFNM.1000269

327. Anand David, A. V., Arulmoli, R., & Parasuraman, S. (2016). Overviews of Biological Importance of Quercetin: A Bioactive Flavonoid. Pharmacognosy reviews, 10(20), 84 89. https://doi.org/10.4103/0973-7847.194044

328. Saeedi-Boroujeni, A., Mahmoudian-Sani, MR. Anti-inflammatory potential of Quercetin in COVID-19 treatment. J Inflamm 18, 3 (2021). https://doi.org/10.1186/s12950-021-00268-6

329. Di Pierro, F., Iqtadar, S., Khan, A., Ullah Mumtaz, S., Masud Chaudhry, M., Bertuccioli, A., Derosa, G., Maffioli, P., Togni, S., Riva, A., Allegrini, P., & Khan, S. (2021). Potential Clinical Benefits of Quercetin in the Early Stage of COVID-19: Results of a Second, Pilot, Randomized, Controlled and Open-Label Clinical Trial. International journal of general medicine, 14, 2807–2816. https://doi.org/10.2147/IJGM.S318949

330. Boretti, A. (2021). Quercetin Supplementation and COVID-19. Natural Product Communications. https://doi.org/10.1177/1934578X211042763

331. : Muhammad F, Ahsan M, Abdul W. Quercetin- A Mini Review. Mod Concep Dev Agrono. 1(2). MCDA.000507. 2018. https://www.researchgate.net/profile/Muhammad-Manzoor-5/publication/332224458_Quercetin-A_Mini_Review/links/5ca7463da6fdcca26dff5fed/Quercetin-A-Mini-Review.pdf?origin=publication_detail

332. Marrelli, M., Amodeo, V., Statti, G., & Conforti, F. (2018). Biological Properties and Bioactive Components of Allium cepa L.: Focus on Potential Benefits in the Treatment of Obesity and Related Comorbidities. Molecules (Basel, Switzerland), 24(1), 119. https://doi.org/10.3390/molecules24010119

333. Nutrition value organization. (n.d.). Onion, raw. Find Nutritional Value of a Product. https://www.nutritionvalue.org/Onions%2C_raw_nutritional_value.html?size=1+cup%2C+chopped+%3D+160+g

334. Tsuboki, J., Fujiwara, Y., Horlad, H., Shiraishi, D., Nohara, T., Tayama, S., Motohara, T., Saito, Y., Ikeda, T., Takaishi, K., Tashiro, H., Yonemoto, Y., Katabuchi, H., Takeya, M., & Komohara, Y. (2016). Onionin A inhibits ovarian cancer progression by suppressing cancer cell proliferation and the protumour function of macrophages. Scientific reports, 6, 29588. https://doi.org/10.1038/srep29588

335. Sharma, K., Mahato, N., & Lee, Y. R. (2018). Systematic study on active compounds as antibacterial and antibiofilm agent in aging onions. Journal of food and drug analysis, 26(2), 518–528. https://doi.org/10.1016/j.jfda.2017.06.009

336. Wang, S., Yao, J., Zhou, B., Yang, J., Chaudry, M. T., Wang, M., Xiao, F., Li, Y., & Yin, W. (2018). Bacteriostatic Effect of Quercetin as an Antibiotic Alternative In Vivo and Its Antibacterial Mechanism In Vitro. Journal of food protection, 81(1), 68–78. https://doi.org/10.4315/0362-028X.JFP-17-214

337. Kumar, V. P., Prashanth, K., & Venkatesh, Y. P. (2015). Structural analyses and immunomodulatory properties of fructo-oligosaccharides from onion (Allium cepa). Carbohydrate polymers, 117, 115–122. https://doi.org/10.1016/j.carbpol.2014.09.039

338. Li, Y., Zheng, X., Yi, X., Liu, C., Kong, D., Zhang, J., & Gong, M. (2017). Myricetin: a potent approach for the treatment of type 2 diabetes as a natural class B GPCR agonist. FASEB journal : official publication of the Federation of American Societies for Experimental Biology, 31(6), 2603–2611. https://doi.org/10.1096/fj.201601339R

339. Ravirajsinh N. Jadeja, Ranjitsinh V. Devkar,Chapter 47 - Polyphenols and Flavonoids in Controlling Non-Alcoholic Steatohepatitis,Editor(s): Ronald Ross Watson, Victor R. Preedy, Sherma Zibadi,

340. Taheri, Y., Suleria, H.A.R., Martins, N. et al. Myricetin bioactive effects: moving from preclinical evidence to potential clinical applications. BMC Complement Med Ther 20, 241 (2020). https://doi.org/10.1186/s12906-020-03033-z

341. Borlinghaus, J., Albrecht, F., Gruhlke, M. C., Nwachukwu, I. D., & Slusarenko, A. J. (2014). Allicin: chemistry and biological properties. Molecules (Basel, Switzerland), 19(8), 12591–12618. https://doi.org/10.3390/molecules190812591

342. Ansary, J., Forbes-Hernández, T. Y., Gil, E., Cianciosi, D., Zhang, J., Elexpuru-Zabaleta, M., Simal-Gandara, J., Giampieri, F., & Battino, M. (2020). Potential Health Benefit of Garlic Based on Human Intervention Studies: A Brief Overview. Antioxidants (Basel, Switzerland), 9(7), 619. https://doi.org/10.3390/antiox9070619

343. Srividya, A. R., Dhanabal, S. P., Misra, V. K., & Suja, G. (2010). Antioxidant and Antimicrobial Activity of Alpinia officinarum. Indian journal of pharmaceutical sciences, 72(1), 145–148. https://doi.org/10.4103/0250-474X.62233

344. Cheah, P. B., & Gan, S. P. (2000). Antioxidative/Antimicrobial effects of galangal and alpha-tocopherol in minced beef. Journal of food protection, 63(3), 404–407. https://doi.org/10.4315/0362-028x-63.3.404

345. Saenghong, N., Wattanathorn, J., Muchimapura, S., Tongun, T., Piyavhatkul, N., Banchonglikitkul, C., & Kajsongkram, T. (2012). Zingiber officinale Improves Cognitive Function of the Middle-Aged Healthy Women. Evidence-based complementary and alternative medicine : eCAM, 2012, 383062. https://doi.org/10.1155/2012/383062

346. Khandouzi, N., Shidfar, F., Rajab, A., Rahideh, T., Hosseini, P., & Mir Taheri, M. (2015). The effects of ginger on fasting blood sugar, hemoglobin a1c, apolipoprotein B, apolipoprotein a-I and malondialdehyde in type 2 diabetic patients. Iranian journal of pharmaceutical research : IJPR, 14(1), 131–140.

347. Kim, Y., Keogh, J. B., & Clifton, P. M. (2016). Polyphenols and Glycemic Control. Nutrients, 8(1), 17. https://doi.org/10.3390/nu8010017

348. Potì, F., Santi, D., Spaggiari, G., Zimetti, F., & Zanotti, I. (2019). Polyphenol Health Effects on Cardiovascular and Neurodegenerative Disorders: A Review and Meta-Analysis. International journal of molecular sciences, 20(2), 351. https://doi.org/10.3390/ijms20020351

349. Chien, S. T., Shi, M. D., Lee, Y. C., Te, C. C., & Shih, Y. W. (2015). Galangin, a novel dietary flavonoid, attenuates metastatic feature via PKC/ERK signaling pathway in TPA-treated liver cancer HepG2 cells. Cancer cell international, 15, 15. https://doi.org/10.1186/s12935-015-0168-2

350. Lo, C. Y., Liu, P. L., Lin, L. C., Chen, Y. T., Hseu, Y. C., Wen, Z. H., & Wang, H. M. (2013). Antimelanoma and antityrosinase from Alpinia galangal constituents. TheScientificWorldJournal, 2013, 186505. https://doi.org/10.1155/2013/186505

351. Song, W., Yan, C. Y., Zhou, Q. Q., & Zhen, L. L. (2017). Galangin potentiates human breast cancer to apoptosis induced by TRAIL through activating AMPK. Biomedicine & pharmacotherapy = Biomedecine & pharmacotherapie, 89, 845–856. https://doi.org/10.1016/j.biopha.2017.01.062

352. Dong, G. Z., Jeong, J. H., Lee, Y. I., Lee, S. Y., Zhao, H. Y., Jeon, R., Lee, H. J., & Ryu, J. H. (2017). Diarylheptanoids suppress proliferation of pancreatic cancer PANC-1 cells through modulating shh-Gli-FoxM1 pathway. Archives of pharmacal research, 40(4), 509–517. https://doi.org/10.1007/s12272-017-0905-2

353. Omoregie, S. N., Omoruyi, F. O., Wright, V. F., Jones, L., & Zimba, P. V. (2013). Antiproliferative activities of lesser galangal (Alpinia officinarum Hance Jam1), turmeric (Curcuma longa L.), and ginger (Zingiber officinale Rosc.) against acute monocytic leukemia. Journal of medicinal food, 16(7), 647–655. https://doi.org/10.1089/jmf.2012.0254

354. Hadjzadeh, M. A., Ghanbari, H., Keshavarzi, Z., & Tavakol-Afshari, J. (2014). The Effects of Aqueous Extract of Alpinia Galangal on Gastric Cancer Cells (AGS) and L929 Cells in Vitro. Iranian journal of cancer prevention, 7(3), 142–146.

355. Zeng, Q. H., Lu, C. L., Zhang, X. W., & Jiang, J. G. (2015). Isolation and identification of ingredients inducing cancer cell death from the seeds of Alpinia galanga, a Chinese spice. Food & function, 6(2), 431–443. https://doi.org/10.1039/c4fo00709c

356. Ha, T. K., Kim, M. E., Yoon, J. H., Bae, S. J., Yeom, J., & Lee, J. S. (2013). Galangin induces human colon cancer cell death via the mitochondrial dysfunction and caspase-dependent pathway. Experimental biology and medicine (Maywood, N.J.), 238(9), 1047–1054. https://doi.org/10.1177/1535370213497882

357. Ghosh, S., & Rangan, L. (2013). Alpinia: the gold mine of future therapeutics. 3 Biotech, 3(3), 173–185. https://doi.org/10.1007/s13205-012-0089-x

358. Srividya, A. R., Dhanabal, S. P., Misra, V. K., & Suja, G. (2010). Antioxidant and Antimicrobial Activity of Alpinia officinarum. Indian journal of pharmaceutical sciences, 72(1), 145–148. https://doi.org/10.4103/0250-474X.62233

359. Altman, R. D., & Marcussen, K. C. (2001). Effects of a ginger extract on knee pain in patients with osteoarthritis. Arthritis and rheumatism, 44(11), 2531–2538. https://doi.org/10.1002/1529-0131(200111)44:11<2531::aid-art433>3.0.co;2-j

360. Lakhan, S. E., Ford, C. T., & Tepper, D. (2015). Zingiberaceae extracts for pain: a systematic review and meta-analysis. Nutrition journal, 14, 50. https://doi.org/10.1186/s12937-015-0038-8

361. Vijayabharathi Rajendiran, Vidhya Natarajan, Sivasithamparam Niranjali Devaraj,

362. Yadav, P. N., Liu, Z., & Rafi, M. M. (2003). A diarylheptanoid from lesser galangal (Alpinia officinarum) inhibits proinflammatory mediators via inhibition of mitogen-activated protein kinase, p44/42, and transcription factor nuclear factor-kappa B. The Journal of pharmacology and experimental therapeutics, 305(3), 925–931. https://doi.org/10.1124/jpet.103.049171

363. Chandrakanthan, M., Handunnetti, S. M., Premakumara, G., & Kathirgamanathar, S. (2020). Topical Anti-Inflammatory Activity of Essential Oils of Alpinia calcarata Rosc., Its Main Constituents, and Possible Mechanism of Action. Evidence-based complementary and alternative medicine : eCAM, 2020, 2035671. https://doi.org/10.1155/2020/2035671

364. Wang, J., Chen, Y., Hu, X., Feng, F., Cai, L., & Chen, F. (2020). Assessing the Effects of Ginger Extract on Polyphenol Profiles and the Subsequent Impact on the Fecal Microbiota by Simulating Digestion and Fermentation In Vitro. Nutrients, 12(10), 3194. https://doi.org/10.3390/nu12103194

365. .T. Mbaveng, V. Kuete,Chapter 30 - Zingiber officinale,Editor(s): Victor Kuete,

366. Maharlouei, N., Tabrizi, R., Lankarani, K. B., Rezaianzadeh, A., Akbari, M., Kolahdooz, F., Rahimi, M., Keneshlou, F., & Asemi, Z. (2019). The effects of ginger intake on weight loss and metabolic profiles among overweight and obese subjects: A systematic review and meta-analysis of randomized controlled trials. Critical reviews in food science and nutrition, 59(11), 1753–1766. https://doi.org/10.1080/10408398.2018.1427044

367. Azam, F., Amer, A. M., Abulifa, A. R., & Elzwawi, M. M. (2014). Ginger components as new leads for the design and development of novel multi-targeted anti-Alzheimer's drugs: a computational investigation. Drug design, development and therapy, 8, 2045–2059. https://doi.org/10.2147/DDDT.S67778

368. USDA. (2011, September). USDA Database for the Flavonoid Content of Selected Foods Release 3. https://www.ars.usda.gov/ARSUserFiles/80400525/Data/Flav/Flav_R03.pdf

369. Chakrawarti, L., Agrawal, R., Dang, S., Gupta, S., & Gabrani, R. (2016). Therapeutic effects of EGCG: a patent review. Expert opinion on therapeutic patents, 26(8), 907–916. https://doi.org/10.1080/13543776.2016.1203419

370. https://www.sciencedirect.com/topics/agricultural-and-biological-sciences/flavanones

371. Kim, J., Wie, M. B., Ahn, M., Tanaka, A., Matsuda, H., & Shin, T. (2019). Benefits of hesperidin in central nervous system disorders: a review. Anatomy & cell biology, 52(4), 369–377. https://doi.org/10.5115/acb.19.119

372. Elzbieta Janda, Antonella Lascala, Concetta Martino, Salvatore Ragusa, Saverio Nucera, Ross Walker, Santo Gratteri, Vincenzo Mollace,Molecular mechanisms of lipid- and glucose-lowering activities of bergamot flavonoids,PharmaNutrition,Volume 4, Supplement,2016,Pages S8-S18,ISSN 2213-4344,

373. Impellizzeri, D., Bruschetta, G., Di Paola, R., Ahmad, A., Campolo, M., Cuzzocrea, S., Esposito, E., & Navarra, M. (2015). The anti-inflammatory and antioxidant effects of bergamot juice extract (BJe) in an experimental model of inflammatory bowel disease. Clinical nutrition (Edinburgh, Scotland), 34(6), 1146–1154. https://doi.org/10.1016/j.clnu.2014.11.012

374. Mandalari, G., Bennett, R., Bisignano, G., Trombetta, D., Saija, A., Faulds, C., Gasson, M. and Narbad, A. (2007), Antimicrobial activity of flavonoids extracted from bergamot (Citrus bergamia Risso) peel, a byproduct of the essential oil industry. Journal of Applied Microbiology, 103: 2056-2064. https://doi.org/10.1111/j.1365-2672.2007.03456.x

375. Bora, H., Kamle, M., Mahato, D. K., Tiwari, P., & Kumar, P. (2020). Citrus Essential Oils (CEOs) and Their Applications in Food: An Overview. Plants (Basel, Switzerland), 9(3), 357. https://doi.org/10.3390/plants9030357

376. Ahmed, Q. U., Ali, A., Mukhtar, S., Alsharif, M. A., Parveen, H., Sabere, A., Nawi, M., Khatib, A., Siddiqui, M. J., Umar, A., & Alhassan, A. M. (2020). Medicinal Potential of Isoflavonoids: Polyphenols That May Cure Diabetes. Molecules (Basel, Switzerland), 25(23), 5491. https://doi.org/10.3390/molecules25235491

377. Miadoková E. (2009). Isoflavonoids - an overview of their biological activities and potential health benefits. Interdisciplinary toxicology, 2(4), 211–218. https://doi.org/10.2478/v10102-009-0021-3

378. Derosa, G., Maffioli, P., & Sahebkar, A. (2016). Ellagic Acid and Its Role in Chronic Diseases. Advances in experimental medicine and biology, 928, 473–479. https://doi.org/10.1007/978-3-319-41334-1_20

379. Amor, A. J., Gómez-Guerrero, C., Ortega, E., Sala-Vila, A., & Lázaro, I. (2020). Ellagic Acid as a Tool to Limit the Diabetes Burden: Updated Evidence. Antioxidants (Basel, Switzerland), 9(12), 1226. https://doi.org/10.3390/antiox9121226

380. Baradaran Rahimi, V., Ghadiri, M., Ramezani, M., & Askari, V. R. (2020). Antiinflammatory and anti-cancer activities of pomegranate and its constituent, ellagic acid: Evidence from cellular, animal, and clinical studies. Phytotherapy research : PTR, 34(4), 685–720. https://doi.org/10.1002/ptr.6565

381. Kang, I., Buckner, T., Shay, N. F., Gu, L., & Chung, S. (2016). Improvements in Metabolic Health with Consumption of Ellagic Acid and Subsequent Conversion into Urolithins: Evidence and Mechanisms. Advances in nutrition (Bethesda, Md.), 7(5), 961–972. https://doi.org/10.3945/an.116.012575

382. Lee, K. H., Jeong, E. S., Jang, G., Na, J. R., Park, S., Kang, W. S., Kim, E., Choi, H., Kim, J. S., & Kim, S. (2020). Unripe Rubus coreanus Miquel Extract Containing Ellagic Acid Regulates AMPK, SREBP-2, HMGCR, and INSIG-1 Signaling and Cholesterol Metabolism In Vitro and In Vivo. Nutrients, 12(3), 610. https://doi.org/10.3390/nu12030610

383. Yang K, Zhang L, Liao P, Xiao Z, Zhang F, Sindaye D, Xin Z, Tan C, Deng J, Yin Y and Deng B (2020) Impact of Gallic Acid on Gut Health: Focus on the Gut Microbiome, Immune Response, and Mechanisms of Action. Front. Immunol. 11:580208. doi:10.3389/fimmu.2020.580208

384. Gao, J., Yang, X., Yin, W., & Li, M. (2018). Gallnuts: A Potential Treasure in Anticancer Drug Discovery. Evidence-based complementary and alternative medicine : eCAM, 2018, 4930371. https://doi.org/10.1155/2018/4930371

385. Alam, M.A., Subhan, N., Hossain, H. et al. Hydroxycinnamic acid derivatives: a potential class of natural compounds for the management of lipid metabolism and obesity. Nutr Metab (Lond) 13, 27 (2016). https://doi.org/10.1186/s12986-016-0080-3

386. Kumar, N., & Pruthi, V. (2014). Potential applications of ferulic acid from natural sources. Biotechnology reports (Amsterdam, Netherlands), 4, 86–93. https://doi.org/10.1016/j.btre.2014.09.002

387. Ronnie J.M. Lubbers, Ronald P. de Vries,Degradation of Homocyclic Aromatic Compounds by Fungi,

388. Allen, R. W., Schwartzman, E., Baker, W. L., Coleman, C. I., & Phung, O. J. (2013). Cinnamon use in type 2 diabetes: an updated systematic review and meta-analysis. Annals of family medicine, 11(5), 452–459. https://doi.org/10.1370/afm.1517

389. Merve Bacanli, Sevtap Aydin Dilsiz, Nurşen Başaran, A. Ahmet Başaran,Chapter Five - Effects of phytochemicals against diabetes,Editor(s): Fidel Toldrá,Advances in Food and Nutrition Research,

390. wikipedia organization. (2021, August 24). Caffeic acid. https://en.wikipedia.org/wiki/Caffeic_acid

391. Shekarchi, M., Hajimehdipoor, H., Saeidnia, S., Gohari, A. R., & Hamedani, M. P. (2012). Comparative study of rosmarinic acid content in some plants of Labiatae family. Pharmacognosy magazine, 8(29), 37–41. https://doi.org/10.4103/0973-1296.93316

392. Kim, G. D., Park, Y. S., Jin, Y. H., & Park, C. S. (2015). Production and applications of rosmarinic acid and structurally related compounds. Applied microbiology and biotechnology, 99(5), 2083–2092. https://doi.org/10.1007/s00253-015-6395-6

393. Al-Dhabi, N. A., Arasu, M. V., Park, C. H., & Park, S. U. (2014). Recent studies on rosmarinic acid and its biological and pharmacological activities. EXCLI journal, 13, 1192–1195.

394. Luo, C., Zou, L., Sun, H., Peng, J., Gao, C., Bao, L., Ji, R., Jin, Y., & Sun, S. (2020). A Review of the Anti-Inflammatory Effects of Rosmarinic Acid on Inflammatory Diseases. Frontiers in pharmacology, 11, 153. https://doi.org/10.3389/fphar.2020.00153

395. Naveed, M., Hejazi, V., Abbas, M., Kamboh, A. A., Khan, G. J., Shumzaid, M., Ahmad, F., Babazadeh, D., FangFang, X., Modarresi-Ghazani, F., WenHua, L., & XiaoHui, Z. (2018). Chlorogenic acid (CGA): A pharmacological review and call for further research. Biomedicine & pharmacotherapy = Biomedecine & pharmacotherapie, 97, 67–74. https://doi.org/10.1016/j.biopha.2017.10.064

396. M. Murkovic,PHENOLIC COMPOUNDS,Editor(s): Benjamin Caballero,Encyclopedia of Food Sciences and Nutrition (Second Edition),Academic Press,2003,Pages 4507-4514,ISBN 9780122270550,

397. Rodríguez-García, C., Sánchez-Quesada, C., Toledo, E., Delgado-Rodríguez, M., & Gaforio, J. J. (2019). Naturally Lignan-Rich Foods: A Dietary Tool for Health Promotion?. Molecules (Basel, Switzerland), 24(5), 917. https://doi.org/10.3390/molecules24050917

398. M.H. Traka,Chapter Nine - Health Benefits of Glucosinolates,Advances in Botanical Research,

399. M.H. Traka,Chapter Nine - Health Benefits of Glucosinolates,Advances in Botanical Research,

400. Alexander, H. (2020, April). SULFORAPHANE BENEFITS: HOW LEAFY VEGGIES LIKE BROCCOLI AND BRUSSELS SPROUTS MAY HELP REDUCE YOUR CANCER RISK. https://www.mdanderson.org/publications/focused-on-health/sulforaphane-benefits--how-leafy-veggies-like-broccoli-and-bruss.h13-1593780.html

401. Fahey, J. W., Zhang, Y., & Talalay, P. (1997). Broccoli sprouts: an exceptionally rich source of inducers of enzymes that protect against chemical carcinogens. Proceedings of the National Academy of Sciences of the United States of America, 94(19), 10367–10372. https://doi.org/10.1073/pnas.94.19.10367

402. Yuanfeng Wu, Yuke Shen, Xuping Wu, Ye Zhu, Jothame Mupunga, Wenna Bao, Jun Huang, Jianwei Mao, Shiwang Liu, and Yuru You. Hydrolysis before Stir-Frying Increases the Isothiocyanate Content of Broccoli, Journal of Agricultural and Food Chemistry 2018 66 (6), 1509-1515. DOI: 10.1021/acs.jafc.7b03913

403. Okunade, O., Niranjan, K., Ghawi, S. K., Kuhnle, G., & Methven, L. (2018). Supplementation of the Diet by Exogenous Myrosinase via Mustard Seeds to Increase the Bioavailability of Sulforaphane in Healthy Human Subjects after the Consumption of Cooked Broccoli. Molecular nutrition & food research, 62(18), e1700980. https://doi.org/10.1002/mnfr.201700980

404. Borgonovo, G., De Petrocellis, L., Schiano Moriello, A., Bertoli, S., Leone, A., Battezzati, A., Mazzini, S., & Bassoli, A. (2020). Moringin, A Stable Isothiocyanate from Moringa oleifera, Activates the Somatosensory and Pain Receptor TRPA1 Channel In Vitro. Molecules (Basel, Switzerland), 25(4), 976. https://doi.org/10.3390/molecules25040976

405. Pandey, K. B., & Rizvi, S. I. (2009). Plant polyphenols as dietary antioxidants in human health and disease. Oxidative medicine and cellular longevity, 2(5), 270–278. https://doi.org/10.4161/oxim.2.5.9498

406. Catalgol, B., Batirel, S., Taga, Y., & Ozer, N. K. (2012). Resveratrol: French paradox revisited. Frontiers in pharmacology, 3, 141. https://doi.org/10.3389/fphar.2012.00141

407. Renaud, S., & de Lorgeril, M. (1992). Wine, alcohol, platelets, and the French paradox for coronary heart disease. Lancet (London, England), 339(8808), 1523–1526. https://doi.org/10.1016/0140-6736(92)91277-f

408. Oregon State University. (n.d.). Resveratrol. Micronutrient Information Center. https://lpi.oregonstate.edu/mic/dietary-factors/phytochemicals/resveratrol

409. Burns, J., Yokota, T., Ashihara, H., Lean, M. E., & Crozier, A. (2002). Plant foods and herbal sources of resveratrol. Journal of agricultural and food chemistry, 50(11), 3337–3340. https://doi.org/10.1021/jf0112973

410. Pérez-Jiménez, J., Neveu, V., Vos, F., & Scalbert, A. (2010). Systematic analysis of the content of 502 polyphenols in 452 foods and beverages: an application of the phenol-explorer database. Journal of agricultural and food chemistry, 58(8), 4959–4969. https://doi.org/10.1021/jf100128b

411. Swetha Salla, Rajitha Sunkara, Simon Ogutu, Lloyd T. Walker, Martha Verghese,

412. Kumoro, A. C., Alhanif, M., & Wardhani, D. H. (2020). A Critical Review on Tropical Fruits Seeds as Prospective Sources of Nutritional and Bioactive Compounds for Functional Foods Development: A Case of Indonesian Exotic Fruits. International journal of food science, 2020, 4051475. https://doi.org/10.1155/2020/4051475

413. Kong, Y. R., Jong, Y. X., Balakrishnan, M., Bok, Z. K., Weng, J., Tay, K. C., Goh, B. H., Ong, Y. S., Chan, K. G., Lee, L. H., & Khaw, K. Y. (2021). Beneficial Role of Carica papaya Extracts and Phytochemicals on Oxidative Stress and Related Diseases: A Mini Review. Biology, 10(4), 287. https://doi.org/10.3390/biology10040287

414. Pérez-Jiménez, J., Neveu, V., Vos, F., & Scalbert, A. (2010). Identification of the 100 richest dietary sources of polyphenols: an application of the Phenol-Explorer database. European journal of clinical nutrition, 64 Suppl 3, S112–S120. https://doi.org/10.1038/ejcn.2010.221

415 Pérez-Jiménez, Jara & Neveu, V & Vos, F & Scalbert, Augustin. (2010). Identification of the 100 richest dietary sources of polyphenols: An application of the Phenol-Explorer database. European journal of clinical nutrition. 64 Suppl 3. S112-20. 10.1038/ejcn.2010.221.

416. Cory, H., Passarelli, S., Szeto, J., Tamez, M., & Mattei, J. (2018). The Role of Polyphenols in Human Health and Food Systems: A Mini-Review. Frontiers in nutrition, 5, 87. https://doi.org/10.3389/fnut.2018.00087

417. da Silveira, M. P., da Silva Fagundes, K. K., Bizuti, M. R., Starck, É., Rossi, R. C., & de Resende E Silva, D. T. (2021). Physical exercise as a tool to help the immune system against COVID-19: an integrative review of the current literature. Clinical and experimental medicine, 21(1), 15–28. https://doi.org/10.1007/s10238-020-00650-3

418. Deemer, S. E., Castleberry, T. J., Irvine, C., Newmire, D. E., Oldham, M., King, G. A., Ben-Ezra, V., Irving, B. A., & Biggerstaff, K. D. (2018). Pilot study: an acute bout of high intensity interval exercise increases 12.5 h GH secretion. Physiological reports, 6(2), e13563. https://doi.org/10.14814/phy2.13563

419. Jiménez-Maldonado, A., Rentería, I., García-Suárez, P. C., Moncada-Jiménez, J., & Freire-Royes, L. F. (2018). The Impact of High-Intensity Interval Training on Brain Derived Neurotrophic Factor in Brain: A Mini-Review. Frontiers in neuroscience, 12, 839. https://doi.org/10.3389/fnins.2018.00839

420. Kim, S. H., & Park, M. J. (2017). Effects of growth hormone on glucose metabolism and insulin resistance in human. Annals of pediatric endocrinology & metabolism, 22(3), 145–152. https://doi.org/10.6065/apem.2017.22.3.145

421. Wisløff, Ulrik1,2; Ellingsen, Øyvind1,2; Kemi, Ole J.3 High-Intensity Interval Training to Maximize Cardiac Benefits of Exercise Training?, Exercise and Sport Sciences Reviews: July 2009 - Volume 37 - Issue 3 - p 139-146 doi: 10.1097/JES.0b013e3181aa65fc

422. Leppäluoto, J., Huttunen, P., Hirvonen, J., Väänänen, A., Tuominen, M., & Vuori, J. (1986). Endocrine effects of repeated sauna bathing. Acta physiologica Scandinavica, 128(3), 467–470. https://doi.org/10.1111/j.1748-1716.1986.tb08000.x

423. Lammintausta, R., Syvälahti, E., & Pekkarinen, A. (1976). Change in hormones reflecting sympathetic activity in the Finnish sauna. Annals of clinical research, 8(4), 266–271.

424. Kukkonen-Harjula, K., Oja, P., Laustiola, K., Vuori, I., Jolkkonen, J., Siitonen, S., & Vapaatalo, H. (1989). Haemodynamic and hormonal responses to heat exposure in a Finnish sauna bath. European journal of applied physiology and occupational physiology, 58(5), 543–550. https://doi.org/10.1007/BF02330710

425. ezová, D., Kvetnanský, R., & Vigas, M. (1994). Sex differences in endocrine response to hyperthermia in sauna. Acta physiologica Scandinavica, 150(3), 293–298. https://doi.org/10.1111/j.1748-1716.1994.tb09689.x

426. Laukkanen T, Khan H, Zaccardi F, Laukkanen JA. Association Between Sauna Bathing and Fatal Cardiovascular and All-Cause Mortality Events. JAMA Intern Med. 2015;175(4):542–548. doi:10.1001/jamainternmed.2014.8187

427. Hannuksela, M. L., & Ellahham, S. (2001). Benefits and risks of sauna bathing. The American journal of medicine, 110(2), 118–126. https://doi.org/10.1016/s0002-9343(00)00671-9

428. Hussain, J., & Cohen, M. (2018). Clinical Effects of Regular Dry Sauna Bathing: A Systematic Review. Evidence-based complementary and alternative medicine : eCAM, 2018, 1857413. https://doi.org/10.1155/2018/1857413

429. Kokura, S., Adachi, S., Manabe, E., Mizushima, K., Hattori, T., Okuda, T., Nakabe, N., Handa, O., Takagi, T., Naito, Y., Yoshida, N., & Yoshikawa, T. (2007). Whole body hyperthermia improves obesity-induced insulin resistance in diabetic mice. International journal of hyperthermia : the official journal of European Society for Hyperthermic Oncology, North American Hyperthermia Group, 23(3), 259–265. https://doi.org/10.1080/02656730601176824

430. Lang, S. A., Moser, C., Fichnter-Feigl, S., Schachtschneider, P., Hellerbrand, C., Schmitz, V., Schlitt, H. J., Geissler, E. K., & Stoeltzing, O. (2009). Targeting heat-shock protein 90 improves efficacy of rapamycin in a model of hepatocellular carcinoma in mice. Hepatology (Baltimore, Md.), 49(2), 523–532. https://doi.org/10.1002/hep.22685

431. Selsby, J. T., Rother, S., Tsuda, S., Pracash, O., Quindry, J., & Dodd, S. L. (2007). Intermittent hyperthermia enhances skeletal muscle regrowth and attenuates oxidative damage following reloading. Journal of applied physiology (Bethesda, Md. : 1985), 102(4), 1702–1707. https://doi.org/10.1152/japplphysiol.00722.2006

432. Scoon, G. S., Hopkins, W. G., Mayhew, S., & Cotter, J. D. (2007). Effect of post-exercise sauna bathing on the endurance performance of competitive male runners. Journal of science and medicine in sport, 10(4), 259–262. https://doi.org/10.1016/j.jsams.2006.06.009

433. Hannuksela, M. L., & Ellahham, S. (2001). Benefits and risks of sauna bathing. The American journal of medicine, 110(2), 118–126. https://doi.org/10.1016/s0002-9343(00)00671-9

434. Pilch, W., Pokora, I., Szyguła, Z., Pałka, T., Pilch, P., Cisoń, T., Malik, L., & Wiecha, S. (2013). Effect of a single finnish sauna session on white blood cell profile and cortisol levels in athletes and non-athletes. Journal of human kinetics, 39, 127–135. https://doi.org/10.2478/hukin-2013-0075

435. Ernst, E., Pecho, E., Wirz, P., & Saradeth, T. (1990). Regular sauna bathing and the incidence of common colds. Annals of medicine, 22(4), 225–227. https://doi.org/10.3109/07853899009148930

436. Masuda, A., Koga, Y., Hattanmaru, M., Minagoe, S., & Tei, C. (2005). The effects of repeated thermal therapy for patients with chronic pain. Psychotherapy and psychosomatics, 74(5), 288–294. https://doi.org/10.1159/000086319

437. Oosterveld, F. G., Rasker, J. J., Floors, M., Landkroon, R., van Rennes, B., Zwijnenberg, J., van de Laar, M. A., & Koel, G. J. (2009). Infrared sauna in patients with rheumatoid arthritis and ankylosing spondylitis. A pilot study showing good tolerance, short-term improvement of pain and stiffness, and a trend towards long-term beneficial effects. Clinical rheumatology, 28(1), 29–34. https://doi.org/10.1007/s10067-008-0977-y

438. Matsumoto, S., Shimodozono, M., Etoh, S., Miyata, R., & Kawahira, K. (2011). Effects of thermal therapy combining sauna therapy and underwater exercise in patients with fibromyalgia. Complementary therapies in clinical practice, 17(3), 162–166. https://doi.org/10.1016/j.ctcp.2010.08.004

439. Fukui, K., Kimura, S., Kato, Y., & Kohno, M. (2021). Effects of far infrared light on Alzheimer's disease-transgenic mice. PloS one, 16(6), e0253320. https://doi.org/10.1371/journal.pone.0253320

440. Dokladny, K., Myers, O. B., & Moseley, P. L. (2015). Heat shock response and autophagy--cooperation and control. Autophagy, 11(2), 200–213. https://doi.org/10.1080/15548627.2015.1009776

441. Chen, S. F., Kang, M. L., Chen, Y. C., Tang, H. W., Huang, C. W., Li, W. H., Lin, C. P., Wang, C. Y., Wang, P. Y., Chen, G. C., & Wang, H. D. (2012). Autophagy-related gene 7 is downstream of heat shock protein 27 in the regulation of eye morphology, polyglutamine toxicity, and lifespan in Drosophila. Journal of biomedical science, 19(1), 52. https://doi.org/10.1186/1423-0127-19-52

442. Benjamin D Horne, Joseph B Muhlestein, Jeffrey L Anderson, Health effects of intermittent fasting: hormesis or harm? A systematic review, The American Journal of Clinical Nutrition, Volume 102, Issue 2, August 2015, Pages 464–470, https://doi.org/10.3945/ajcn.115.109553

443. Zhengxiang Huang, Lili Huang, Michael J. Waters, Chen Chen,Insulin and Growth Hormone Balance: Implications for Obesity,Trends in Endocrinology & Metabolism,Volume 31, Issue 9,2020,Pages 642-654,

444. Mohammad Bagheriya, Alexandra E. Butler, George E. Barreto, Amirhossein Sahebkar,

445. Johnstone, A. Fasting for weight loss: an effective strategy or latest dieting trend?. Int J Obes 39, 727–733 (2015). https://doi.org/10.1038/ijo.2014.214

446. Adrienne R. Barnosky, Kristin K. Hoddy, Terry G. Unterman, Krista A. Varady,

447. Adrienne R. Barnosky, Kristin K. Hoddy, Terry G. Unterman, Krista A. Varady,

448. Aftab Ahmed, Farhan Saeed, Muhammad Umair Arshad, Muhammad Afzaal, Ali Imran, Shinawar Waseem Ali, Bushra Niaz, Awais Ahmad & Muhammad Imran (2018) Impact of intermittent fasting on human health: an extended review of metabolic cascades, International Journal of Food Properties, 21:1, 2700-2713, DOI: 10.1080/10942912.2018.1560312

449. Mattson, M., Moehl, K., Ghena, N. et al. Intermittent metabolic switching, neuroplasticity and brain health. Nat Rev Neurosci 19, 81–94 (2018). https://doi.org/10.1038/nrn.2017.156

ABOUT THE AUTHOR

Triya Redberg is a Certified Nutrition Consultant; specializing in blood sugar stabilization. She has been working in the health & fitness field as a personal trainer, yoga instructor, and group class instructor for over 15 years. She holds certifications from the National Academy of Sports Medicine (NASM), the International Sports Science Association (ISSA), and the International Fitness Professionals Association (IFPA).

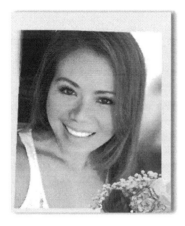

She won bodybuilder shows in Northern California and practices what she preaches;

Credentials

• 2nd place Figure class B, NPC Bodybuilding, Figure, Bikini, Fitness, San Jose Championships 2009

• 4th place Master Bikini class A, Bodybuilding, Figure, Bikini, Fitness, Costa Championships 2011

• 2nd place Master Bikini class A, Bodybuilding, Figure, Bikini, Fitness, San Francisco Championships 2011

• 5th place Open Bikini Class C, Bodybuilding, Figure, Bikini, Fitness, San Francisco Championships 2011

Triya holds a B.A. in Arts from Silpakorn University, one of the top 5 universities in Thailand. She cherishes art, productive projects, and enthusiasm for learning new things and advancing her knowledge. She holds certifications in digital media and design from the University of Connecticut and Multimedia from City College of San Francisco.

Triya embodies a holistic approach to healing and living. Her passion is to educate and assist her clients to integrate successful and enjoyable; healthy eating and wellness experiences. And most of all, for them to be easy and sustainable!

Apart from fitness and nutrition, she also has a solid knowledge of Ayurveda, herbal remedies, essential oils, massage therapy, and a licensed massage therapist.

Triya was born and raised in Thailand, has been living in the United States since 2001, and she is a Hawaiian resident since 2014.